Every Day a Little Miracle

Kirsten Kuhnert

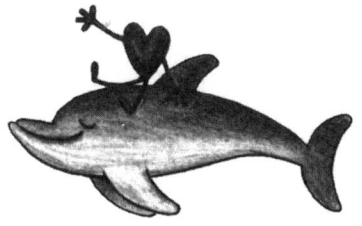

The Gift of The Dolphins

Smart Publishing

© 2002 Smart Publishing Pty Ltd

First published 1999 by Wilhelm Heyne Verlag GmbH & Co. KG. München
English edition 2002 by Smart Publishing Pty Ltd

Offices:	Australia:
	PO Box 1340
	Noosaville DC, QLD 4566
	Europe:
	Goethering 48
	63303 Dreieich, Germany
	USA:
	260 Crandon Blvd
	Suite 32-147,
	Key Biscayne, FL 33149
	http://www.dolphins-miracle.com
	info@dolphins-miracle.com
Produced by:	CopyRight Publishing Brisbane Australia
Printed by:	Watson Ferguson & C° Brisbane
Translation by:	Tony Martin and Kirsten Kuhnert from the German original
Cover design by:	esdesign, Sebastian Rothe
Photographs by:	Nomi Baumgartl, Constanze Wild and Markus Tedeskino

All rights reserved. No part of this publication may be reproduced, stored in a retrieval system, or transmitted in any form or by any means, electronic, mechanical, photocopying, recording or otherwise, without the prior permission of the Publisher.

ISBN   1 876344 10 5 Hard cover
       1 876344 11 3 Soft cover

Contents

Foreword by HRH Prinz Leopold von Bayern   7

I   Timmy — an extraordinary story   9
Timmy's story 11 • The tragedy 14 • The endless trail through clinics — our odyssey 24 • Friends 34 • Therapy — What is it? 43 • Doctors, healers and 'quacks' 48 • Our family grows: Timmy's care team 57 • The first contact with Dolphin Human Therapy 65 • Dr Nathanson and his team 76 • Timmy's first trip to the dolphins 84 • The value of hope 105 • Spunky, a very special dolphin 112 • Quite normal madness 118 • A charity grows 127 • The present 147 • The darker side 160 • Joy 165 • A journey through time 169 • Today is Yesterday's Future 178 • How is Timmy 182 • Success arises ... 185 • Exactly how does Dolphin Human Therapy work 192

II   The dolphins help many children   195
A word from Dr David E. Nathanson 197 • What is Dolphin Human Therapy? 198 • How does one describe a 'dream job'? 205 • Dolphin therapy, a bird's-eye view 207 • A big success 212 • Lukas 213 • Katharina 217 • Alexandra 220 • Nadia 222 • Kristina 226 • Cindy 229

III   *Addendum*   235
What is dolphin aid? 237 • The aims of the charity 240 • The therapy centres 241 • Glossary 243 • Some helpful addresses for the parents of sick and 'special needs' children 244 • My thanks 246 • Nomi Baumgartl 251

For Tim and Kira

In the Memory of Maurice, Christian,
Sebastian, Prisca-Kim, Timo and Maxi

Foreword by HRH Prinz Leopold von Bayern

We all know people who never recover from blows dealt by fate. Giving up, they die slowly even if their bodies are still working fine. Many don't even think it is possible to come to terms with their predicament.

Kirsten Kuhnert, the author of this book, did not give up when she experienced a cruel stroke of fate several years ago. Rather than resign herself to accepting an unacceptable outcome, she called up unimaginable inner strength to not only help her son through his traumatic experience, but she has helped so many others, supporting them through similar situations in which she found herself.

My friend of many years Kirsten Kuhnert writes the story of her life and that of her children, especially her son, handicapped by a near-drowning accident, with remarkable openness and honesty. She reveals much of herself and her innermost thoughts with admirable frankness.

This book is far more than just a descriptive message. It is one of the very special books in my life. It gives hope and the desire to confront each and every imaginable personal situation and to enable people to learn to cope with it.

She shows that having the strength to go forward and the power to open each and every new door is the only chance to survive, in the certainty that beyond these doors a new opportunity waits. Kirsten Kuhnert has thrown open many such doors. Some opened easier than others, and for some she needed all her strength – but open them all she did!

Kirsten Kuhnert's first trip to the dolphins was most certainly the beginning of a fabulous journey, a story of many little miracles. Besides giving others who were not as strong as herself a helping hand, she raised millions of dollars to support research and to help over 700 children experience the wonders of Human Dolphin Therapy.

This book will open your eyes to a fascinating experience. It is written for all of us, those who are lucky, healthy and in good shape, and those who are not as lucky, desperate people and troubled families coping with injured and handicapped dependants.

HRH Prinz Leopold von Bayern[1]

---

[1] *Also known as His Royal Highness Prince Leopold of Bavaria*

I

Timmy — An Extraordinary Story

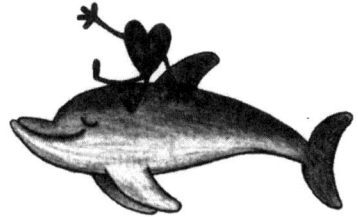

Timmy's story

This is really Timmy's story. Of course at the present time he is not in the position to tell it himself. For Timmy cannot speak. Neither can he walk, or romp about, or play with other kids in the sandpit. But he is there, and that in itself is a miracle.

So I stroke him gently, when I sense that he needs me near to him; I told him what I saw when his eyes could not see the world around him; I scratch him, sensing he has an itch; I tell him that one day he will be healthy again; and so will I tell his story, for this too is my story. It is the story of a very special boy who is very brave and who has also taught me courage. On his long journey this little guy, my son, has made wonderful things happen, has changed many people's points of view and, in spite of endless worries, has made my life so much richer.

Tim's story is a story of survival, survival for everyone in every possible situation.

During his first meeting with Spunky the lady dolphin, a little miracle occurred — Tim laughed heartily, and was happy — for the first time, almost a year and a half after his accident. From this indescribable feeling of joy I reached the decision to found an organization which would make it possible for other handicapped children to have a therapeutic meeting with the dolphins. Suddenly I had more than two thousand god-children!!!!

No story is the same as another, each family copes differently with the demands of these 'special children'. Often, with very mixed emotions, I read the letters of hoping, dedicated but also despairing people.

I can feel their pain, and I sense their will and strength in trying to overcome their problems, in seeking paths for their 'special children' to a better quality of life.

From these personal stories I gain the strength and motivation to continue with this highly complex and energy consuming project for Timmy and all the other little ones who especially need our help.

Furthermore following Tim's accident I would have been so pleased if an organisation like *dolphin aid* already existed — simply as a place to turn to with questions, troubles, fears and for a little hope.

Like Timmy, each of these *dolphin aid* kids is unique, like Timmy, each of these children has a personal, incomparable story.

Nevertheless there are certain things that they all have in common. These children show their parents that they have more strength in them than they had ever imagined possible, and teach that one is able to bear far more than one had ever thought, in the knowledge of being needed so much. They show us that it is possible to far exceed the previously accepted boundaries of nervous strength, with the best available source of energy available in this world — Love.

I was gifted and blessed with the chance of meeting several of my 'god-children' personally.

They all impressed me — as outstanding characters. Irrespective how great the degree of their momentary 'handicap' may be, they have brought about much. They have changed the points of view of those around them, set different standards, have not only created 'plans for life' but often changed them, they have opened the eyes of so many people, and with this, have forced their environment to concentrate on elementary values. Each of these little BIG kids means a lot to me and I am very happy that I was able to meet them.

Tim's story is the story of *dolphin aid*. Tim is dolphin aid. And I tell the story of my son with the unshakeable hope that one day we will, together with his little sister Kira and several other special people, reach the end of a very long path, and he will be able to say whether all my emotions, fears and dreams showed us the right way.

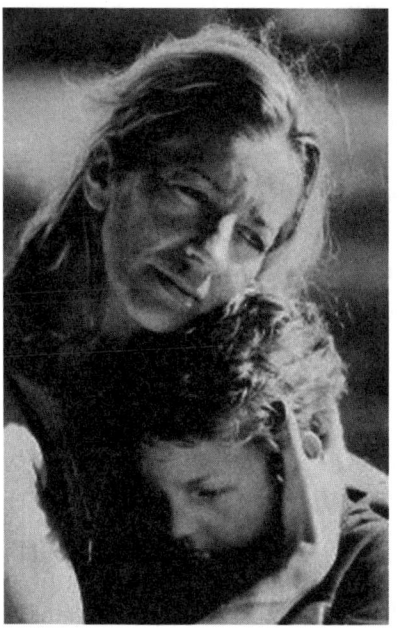

Tim and Kiki

The Tragedy

Timmy is a child of the Sun. On the day on which he chose to become part of this life, the sun was shining, on the day of his birth the sun was shining, and also on that fateful day of his accident the sun shone too, the christening day of his little sister Kira. Sunshine was always something especially important for Timmy and also today it gives him the necessary strength to master his difficult path until such time when he may be a normal young boy again.

Tim was a wanted child, a wished for and loved child. A quite special child. Each and every Mother thinks that her child is special, and so it is that each, in his or her own particular way, is quite unique. What is then the progression, the heightening of this 'special'?

Tim had an aura which simply radiated and charmed even the most hardened people who weren't very fond of children, a magic which, together with his personality simply gathered everyone forever under his own personal spell.

I conceived him and he was born as the greatest gift in my life, and yet I had this feeling, from the beginning, that he would be taken away from me. I will always remember the shocked expression on my Mother's face as I told her this. She asked that I should never repeat these thoughts ever again, and later she was to remember herself these words in the most painful circumstances.

Many of the people we meet today, when they look at Tim, say such absurd things like 'How terrible, while he is such a beautiful child'. As if it was of such importance whether a child is beautiful or not! But these absurd remarks prove that Tim, even though he cannot behave like other children, has lost none of his magic.

Timmy is now nine years old, and when I see how gloriously his sister is developing, her pleasure in exploring everything, see how she can break down every barrier with her childish logic, know how wonderful it is to laugh together with her, to look at the stars together and perceive the entire world as one huge miracle — it is at such times that I feel, without just feeling sorry for myself, that I have been betrayed these experiences with Timmy.

The memories of this wonderful normality ended for myself and my son on 18 June 1994 — the day of Kira's baptism. Up until this date our lives, at least on the outside, ran perfectly. Two wonderful children, first a son and then twenty-one months later a daughter, exactly as things should be. My father-in-law provided us with a villa on the edge of town, and how we lived inside was nobody else's business.

It was a mark of our status that the ladies wore hats as we celebrated the baptism at a golf club, with a small circle of family and friends. From the wonderful sermon of the pastor right through to the very amusing speech given by Kira's godfather, all was filmed for posterity on video. The guests all proceeded outside onto the terrace, and, against our usual habit, my husband and I withdrew from the others so that we could read a letter from my father-in-law and some of the congratulatory telegrams, safe in the knowledge that the children were in the good hands and protection of the family and close friends.

The newly-lit cigarette did not survive three puffs, and from one second to the next Timmy was no longer there.

It is so hard to continue at this point, the fear and paralyzing knowledge that something terrible had happened takes hold of me, and it is as if I am forced once again to relive those horrifying moments. The breathless search, the cries, my imploring, reaching a screaming climax, and finally, from a long distance the picture of my beloved son being lifted out of the 'damned' pool and the lifeless bundle being carried away. With my cry to Martin, a doctor friend 'who must make everything right again', I took leave of all conscious thought for a very long time.

I see my drowned, lifeless child lying there, but it is not Tim. I speak, call to him, wherever he now is. 'Breathe, you must breathe, Timmy do you hear? breathe ... Stay here, you must stay by Mami, Timmy you **must** breathe, come back to Mami, Timmy breathe, my child, my beloved listen to Mami, do you hear me you **must** breathe ...'

My mother's face appears, but it is not her face, it is a mask, she too is dead from the dreadful shock.

Tim's father, my husband Jack, has collapsed against the wall of a house. Why? He is crying, he must stop whining and whinging he must talk to his son!! Tim

must breathe 'Do you hear what Mami says? Timmy you must breathe, breathe my child ...'

They do not let me go to my child, but this is not so important as that which lies there is not my child. I must get Timmy back from wherever he has gone, he must be re-united with that which is lying there.

The emergency ambulance is not there! Later I learnt that it took almost twenty-five minutes. I don't care. I hardly register this information, I speak to my son over and over, without end.

People try to hold me, touch me — I don't want to be touched — I only want my child back. I am alone. I don't know where Timmy's father is. He doesn't talk to his son. He suffers. He should do something instead of just sitting there and crying. I must get Timmy back.

Timmy is lying in the ambulance — I creep past — hear heartbeats at last — but I am not really calmed by this — just a small victory, no relief — disjointed, scrambled parts of sentences over the ambulance radio. 'There is no intensive-care bed at the clinic — Do you hear? — over.' What are they talking about, my child doesn't need a bed, my child must live!!!

'St George's Memorial could take him — what about the helicopter?'

Timmy is breathing again. I don't want him to fly alone, but the helicopter is not big enough. My husband and father-in-law drive off in advance so that someone is there to meet Timmy at the clinic.

I have to wait until the helicopter with Timmy takes off.

And then, in my uncle's car I follow the helicopter carrying my son, my baby, to the clinic. I am very surprisingly collected. I am smoking one of Kay's non-filter cigarettes, I don't have any of my own. I feel sick, I'm falling ... all becomes clear to me; Kira my little princess, my 'Püppi', my little one — just four months old, will never want for anything, nor could there be anything she could miss. I truly love her from the bottom of my heart, but there is no doubt at all that if they tell me at the hospital that there is nothing more they can do for my son, I know that I will never want to go home again!!

The clinic is close to the High School where I spent most of my school years. I hated it, and I always felt compulsively unwell here. I have not been here for ages. I never wanted to be in this town. What an irony that on this day I have to return.

People, many people, are standing around at the entrance to the Intensive-Care Unit. I no longer know how many or who they were. I want to be with my child — it cannot be good when I am not at his side.

The doctor in charge of the Intensive-Care Unit, Dr Ibach is an understanding man. 'That which we have to do here with your child is known as "craftsmanship" which any doctor on the Intensive-Care Unit must be able to deal with. The deciding factor for us is the state in which we receive the little patient, and there are three indications which are of paramount importance:-

1. The heart function
2. Unaided breathing
3. Constant pupil eye reaction to light.

'In my own personal experience, and in the present medical situation your son will leave this clinic with a 95% chance of being in the same condition he was in before falling into the old pool' ... and in a very small voice he continued ... 'for the other 5% we are on the outside looking in. This is in Gods hands.'

All of those gathered breathe easier, by cell phones the news is broadcast to friends. A man, who I don't even know, puts his arms around me and cries for happiness and relief. I want to be with my child. It cannot be right that I am not with him. I am far away from any relief — I am filled with fear.

As I was clothed in a blue Intensive-Care overall, I notice for the first time that I had no shoes — I had no idea how long I have been walking barefoot. A nursing sister gave me OP shoes.

At last, at long last, I am with my son. He looks so terribly pale, deathly pale. I stroke him, he is as cold as ice 'Why, why', I ask. Dr Ibach regarded me for a long time. The monitor shows Tim's body temperature 28.9^0 C. He was dead, but now he lives again!

Slowly, I hope, with the increase in his body temperature, life will return into his beloved little body, he will open his eyes and say something like 'Mami, Tinny must sleep in big bed', and all will be well again!!

Today I cannot even tell with any degree of certainty what I really felt at this moment or if I knew, or guessed, that Ibach was deceiving himself in thinking that everything was 'not so bad'.

The first MRT result does not show any significant damage, at least that's what they tell me. Now I begin to breathe a little easier, at least a very little, but Timmy is still in coma. Dr Ibach is perplexed, at a loss, we discuss over and over, day and night, various theories why Timmy does not regain consciousness. We lay his sister naked on his belly, we bring the dog, his dog to the hospital, I spread his much-loved ketchup on his tongue, everything — anything — in the desperate hope that these intimate, familiar experiences may call him back from the coma.

Except for only a few addictive puffs on a cigarette, I never leave my child alone. The first nights I spend in a rocking chair by his bed. On the morning of the fifth day Timmy called suddenly, loud and very clearly '**Mami**'.

I am as if paralyzed. 'Mami is here, Timmy, Mami is with you.' He doesn't react. I think I am going crazy. 'Timmy, you called me, I am here, with you — please speak to me.' Nothing.

Did I dream it? I am totally desperate. Sister Susanne looks carefully at me — I'm not crazy — and then she says, 'I heard it too, and I will say so even if they then think I have gone mad'.

To date that was the last time that I really actually heard Timmy speak.

From this point in time onwards we shared the Intensive-Care bed at night. It was no longer enough for me to just hold his hand. I needed to feel his entire body and to give him my warmth — the warmth and love that only a mother can give. I guarded his deceptive sleep so that I should not miss even the slightest movement.

With every single fibre of my body and with all my love I hoped that he might give me some small sign, some small indication that might reduce my fear.

Instead of this, after a few days, 'extreme pathological symptoms' set in, which led to the conclusion that in his beautiful little head something must have been destroyed, and that this, at least for a very long time, would prevent things from being the way they were before.

For almost two weeks I did not cry one single tear. Fully grown men such as my uncle stood at Timmy's bedside in tears, overcome with emotion as I remained, day in and day out, night after night, upright and almost empty of emotion.

When I finally lost control and broke down in floods of tears, everyone was relieved. Everyone on the ward crowded together to say, 'At last, we thought we would have to send you to a psychiatric hospital'.

It was good to be held by so many loving and caring people who also spoke to me in the kindest ways, knowing in their own hearts that not one single word of that which they said could help me.

But the honest kindness combined with the interest and devotional care will never ever be forgotten by me — they all have my deepest thanks.

In the following days Timmy began groaning, he sweated profusely, and his little body was gripped with spasms, his limbs took on grotesque directions — and nevertheless he was taken from the Intensive-Care Unit and put onto a normal nursing ward.

I had the feeling that we had become homeless. I had never imagined that I would wish again for the security of an Intensive-Care Unit.

My whole existence was composed only of fear and anxiety.

Dr Ibach made it clear to me that from the therapeutic point of view there was nothing further they could do here for Tim, and that he must be transferred to another hospital. He would give us time to consider, but how could we decide which hospital? Mentally and physically strained, we had no idea, absolutely no idea, what was important or necessary for Timmy from a medical point of view.

In the meantime Timmy's bed in the Intensive-Care Unit was now occupied by another young boy who had also suffered from a drowning accident. He died. I noted this fact but I honestly cannot tell truly what I felt, or whether I felt anything at all.

I am often asked how, or whether, I have mentally been able to overcome and digest Timmy's accident.

The answer to this is — so far, not at all!!

Most people then think that I need psychological help. What a false conclusion! If I were to put myself on the couch now, I would probably not ever get up again! There will be time for all that when Timmy one day will be able to take care of himself again, and Kira's natural growth and healthy development will give me the energy to simply let go.

Sometimes, however, I wish that I was able, and could allow myself, to say, 'I cannot manage any more, and I don't want to any more, please just call my Mother'. But such short periods of weakness follow long periods of stubborn and defiant strength after the motto 'I am not going to let this thing beat me, or beat us! We have managed up to now, and so we continue — the way is forward'.

I am often also asked where I get the strength. To tell the truth I don't know myself sometimes, I really don't know exactly. The strength is just there, I have to be strong, and my values and visions of the future help me to see it through. What I do know, however, is 'Love can conquer all'. If you give love, more is coming back to you than you give away.

Timmy presents me with a very hard test. Three steps forward and then five steps backwards; each little success, each tiny glimmer of hope about Timmy's condition I have had to pay for many times over in seemingly endless despair or disappointment. Even so I have never, in the remotest corner of my mind, truly thought of giving up, even though at times there may have been simpler solutions.

My son has shown me that I have greater strength in me than I ever could have imagined, so it is that I have simply retained my strength and I have not given up.

Although many situations in the time since Timmy's accident have certainly given me cause to lose my balance, it was always clear to me in my mind that both my children need me.

Of course there were phases when I counted the stock of Valium in our household, when I said to myself that would be enough; and I am not ashamed to admit that there were also moments, when I could not, and did not want to, bear the pain any longer. I wanted to be freed from all of that which shook my body with vomiting cramps. Yes, sometimes I have thought 'That's enough', and with the thought 'Whatever have I done to deserve all this?' very nearly capitulated. Painfully, I have had to learn to deal with these depressive phases, but I never lost from view my single aim which has the name — Timmy's recovery! And that still costs enormous effort and we still have a long way to go.

The endless trail through clinics — our odyssey

Even before Timmy was born we decided upon medical examinations which would show whether we were expecting a normal, healthy child.

A very close friend of mine, one year previously, had given birth to a severely handicapped child and both my husband and I wanted to be certain that this would not happen to us. We had given, however, absolutely no thought to how we would react to such an event.

Spontaneously and with unusual unity we both replied to the doctor's questions as to how we would deal with something like this happening. We didn't feel capable of raising a sick child. Suddenly no-one asked such questions any more.

Timmy was not just a 'cared-for' child. You could really almost say that he was guarded. Our house was like a fortress, for a child, with every safety factor. And nevertheless it happened, my worst nightmare, my horror visions became the dreadful reality.

And nothing from our experience or knowledge, none of our energy or activity could do anything to change Timmy's condition. Suddenly we had to make decisions, the scope of which we had not the slightest idea. We fought with medical diagnoses which we did not even understand. And why, if you please could no-one tell us what to do??

Dr Ibach made it crystal clear to us that the time had arrived to have Timmy transferred to a specialist clinic. This was a terrible thought because I felt at least safe in this Children's Hospital.

This good man had become for me a trusted and important person. We spoke together for hours on end about Timmy's condition. Even he, the experienced doctor, was puzzled and despondent about the way things were going with Timmy.

His words remain in my mind to this day — 'With a 95% chance your son will leave the clinic in the same condition he was in before falling into the pool'. He seemed so sure of himself, but in the end it was that 5% 'that only heaven knows', which was to be our fate.

I will always have a picture of this doctor in my mind. I think of him with great affection, his wide-awake eyes which observed me with a mixture of intelligence and trust-evoking human warmth. This doctor was most important to me in the months following Tim's accident. And today in moments of helplessness I stick to things he told me.

There must have been something that made him think that Timmy would again become healthy.

Dr Ibach, this combination of a sympathetic father-like friend and the absent-minded professor now wished to arrange for Tim to be transferred to another hospital. Each day we discussed, in Timmy's room, what was the next step which would be right for him. Rehabilitation or University clinic? Bobath[1], Votja[1], Sensory Integration, a stomach probe through the abdominal wall ? — and of all these things I had not the slightest understanding.

Martin Schata, Tim's lifesaver, an allergy specialist, was not exactly specialized for a brain-damaged little accident victim. In the time since the accident he had occupied himself almost fulltime questioning all his colleagues and informing himself what the best form of care would be for Timmy and where to obtain this care. Almost every day he came to visit us in the clinic. Tim became much more for him than just the child of his friends. During the half hour of reanimation, he had given of himself in a dimension above the normal human being. He gave Timmy the gift of life for the second time.

Timmy's grandfather, my father-in-law, the indisputable 'Head of the Family' almost died inwardly on his situation of helpless impotence.

He, too, contacted all possible sources in the hope that they could offer some help. In the end it was destiny that was to decide, following our endless discussions, into which clinic my son would be transferred. A friend of my father-in-law was the chairman of the clinical board of a large neurological children's clinic not far away. With the help of his connections it was guaranteed that Timmy was transferred there as not being 'just a number'.

It was very hard for both of us to take leave of Dr Ibach and his team of helpers on the intensive care unit. They had given us security and the assurance that in the days following the accident someone was always at my side when I was consumed by anxiety and fears.

[1] Forms of therapy

Because Timmy was only partially fit for travel, Dr Ibach arranged a helicopter. The flight took place with almost complete silence between us. It seemed as if it was painful for him to give the care of his little patient, whom he had accompanied through the first dark nights, into the hands of someone else. We assured one another that we would remain in constant contact. I held Timmy's hand and felt lost — lost beyond comprehension.

The following days and weeks in the new clinic were pure hell. Timmy's condition deteriorated almost by the hour. He sighed and groaned and choked. He sweated and his heart raced like a madman's. As if hypnotized, I stared at the monitors by day and night whilst holding my child in my arms. In the night we shared his little bed. Timmy's pulse rate rose to unbelievable heights, and there were times when I thought that his little heart would jump out of his chest! His reaction to calming drugs was that he became even more agitated.

With Martin's assistance, and the assurance that a doctor would be permanently on hand, Timmy and I were, after two months, allowed for the first time to spend a weekend at home. I could hardly wait to have my little daughter, who was in the care of my mother, for myself — for a whole weekend. Her short visits to the clinic were no substitute and I had such a longing to be near her. I wanted to stroke her and for her to fall asleep in my arms. In the deepest part of my soul I hoped that, after a while, the only remaining feeling about the accident would be that I had left my little girl alone for too long.

From our next weekend break we were never to return to this clinic.

From what I know today it was almost irresponsible to take my son home, without equipment and any special knowledge, merely the unbelievably strong desire for a semblance of normality, but with the unbounded belief that in his accustomed surroundings he would be better.

Many times in the night when Timmy's fight against his own body caused screams and crying, shaken with spasms, and when his temperature soared to well over 40^0 C, we had to call for Martin. How many times was I as if paralysed and didn't know how to continue???

And so it was that at regular intervals we found ourselves in various hospitals, in which very often I had to fear once more for Tim's life, for his problems were, most of the times, beyond their capabilities.

At the end of the day was always the recognition that we were both absolutely alone and therefore best off at home. Anxiety and fear remained our constant companions.

The stay in a clinic of alternative medicine, in which we had placed such high hopes in their enthusiasm, only resulted in a deterioration in Tim. They had tried, some days, up to five different forms of therapy. The only things that calmed him to any degree at all were body-contact and gentle rocking motions with my body and legs, while he sat in my lap. It became clearer and clearer that Timmy's condition would not improve in a hospital.

After two months I was able to give him liquids, foods and medicines via a nasal tube to his stomach and I had been able to motivate him into swallowing with the help of a syringe, drop by drop. I was prepared to do anything in order to make it possible for him to have, at home, any imaginable rehabilitation measures.

In all the weeks and months of our ever-repeated visits to clinics, we came into contact with many nurses and therapists.

Looking back I can only say that those who remain in my mind with positive memory following our 'Intensive-care times' can be counted on one hand. But for a few exceptions no one expressed any understanding for the anxieties and fears or for the desperation of a mother. Only too often was I a disturbance in the hospital routine.

For many of the nursing staff I was just someone who 'got on their nerves' with my constant questions, follow ups, reminders and any requests which I had. This feeling was to be a long time companion.

Even today I am 'allergic' to the impatient look, the raised eyebrows, the nasal snorts of the permanently stressed and often arrogant ladies and gentlemen who took up the care and nursing of their fellow human beings, as a profession, of their own free will.

But there were also very special people, who in the very hardest times, with a special understanding, were either at my side or who held me, crying, in their arms — and who after days, weeks and months of restlessness tried to order me to go and sleep; people who tried to give me comfort and consolation, knowing that in my situation consolation was impossible; people who gave me courage; people who gave me valuable and sometimes the deciding, or at the end, life-saving ideas; people who gave me advice, and those who, with sincerity, shared with me the fears for the life of my son. All of these people with their admirable help did much to make this time 'survivable'. I feel a great bond with them and I hope with all my heart that one day Timmy may be able also to thank all of them personally.

In this time of helplessness I got to know a very special doctor: Dr Michael Mandl, a child neurologist at the University Clinic, Düsseldorf. Following our endless journey through various hospitals and clinics it was in the end Dr Mandl who became Timmy's 'personal' doctor. Still, today, I am so grateful in this choice for my son; we both have found in Dr Mandl someone who is both a friend and reliable partner. It is thanks to this extraordinary man alone that even today Timmy shows no fear when he goes to give blood for tests, for the several hundredth time. From the first day of the dreadful diagnosis *Status Epilepticus* he treated Tim as a buddy. He has been more of a friend to me in terrible situations, than some whom I have known my whole life. After Dr Ibach he was the first person in whom I developed a real trust.

The very thought of putting Timmy in a University Clinic filled me with a determined aversion. I was frightened that they would try to experiment with him or even give him into the hands of less experienced doctors. But then it was that, in the University Clinic, the first and decisive improvement was achieved for my child. After the crushing diagnosis 'epileptic fits' and 'extreme pathological EEG[2]', the doctors at least knew where they had to begin with any therapeutic treatment. Timmy had to be given the appropriate daily dosage of medicines and I can tell you that my vocabulary had to

[2] Electroencephalogram

increase as I had to cope even with the spelling of the term Epilepsy!!

In the meantime it was already November. Five months after this absurd accident my son still could not sleep. He no longer had any day and night cycle, and he fought onward with unseen forces and was just a shadow of the former magical scallywag he once was.

He had lost more than eight pounds in weight and his previously sturdy thighs which simply looked 'good enough to eat' had lost all form, the muscles had deteriorated — his angel-face too was now just a pain-torn mask. You could say that he was reduced to a skeleton. The never-ending battle to pump as many calories into him as possible was the only thing which stopped him losing even more weight.

At this time I was filled with hatred for all doctors, except Dr Mandl, who revolved around Timmy. For no-one else really made any effort at all for my son. No-one could tell me how to reduce the agony of his tortured little body. The worst thing of all was that no-one seemed to have the slightest interest to reduce this inhuman suffering. When Dr Mandl was not present, there were constant excessive medical discussions with doctors against whose human and professional incapability I felt utterly defenceless.

It happened during the visit of one of the head doctors, with his procession of followers, that I finally exploded and told him exactly what I thought about the present situation. I was no longer willing to accept that when I rang for help in the night it sometimes took up to an hour for anyone to come, and then to be asked

'What's the problem — What, you again! — What do you expect us to do' and other such foolish remarks, while I held in my arms a cramp-ridden, screaming bundle whose pulse often raced at the rate of two hundred and twenty!!!

I made it clear about my suspicions that here nothing further would be achieved. In fact I told them of my certainty that at home, with an emergency in the night, help would be available much faster if I called the ambulance and emergency doctor to the house, and that way return Timmy to the clinic as an emergency case. Everybody present seemed visibly shocked.

For several seconds there was complete silence, and when I heard the decisive voice of ward-sister Hildegard 'Now just listen to me Mrs Kuhnert', I was ready for the offensive. But as I listened carefully, her words were astonishing. 'All nurses and staff are on your side — this situation cannot go on. This child must sleep at last and something positive must happen. If things carry on as they are, Timmy will only get worse and the two of you would not survive that.'

That certainly 'gave me one back'. They all withdrew and I sat with Timmy in my arms, on that hospital bed, and for the first time in ages, felt something which was a little like relief. Obviously there really were people who did not just think that I was a hysterical mother who did not want to accept her fate. Suddenly there was someone who took me seriously and spoke out on that for which I was hoping.

One hour later I was told by the professor that he had decided to give Timmy a newly developed medicine, from which they hoped he would benefit. It at least might give him the much hoped-for peace at night.

That night Timmy slept, for the first time in almost six months. With disbelief and also with fear I constantly felt his pulse to assure myself that he really was still alive. The fact he really was sleeping seemed to me to be almost abnormal, and at some stage I too must have fallen asleep — Timmy's hand in mine.

Hours later I awoke in total confusion, and close to a heart-attack in those first seconds thinking that Timmy was dead. Then the tears just streamed over my cheeks as I saw my beloved child breathing easily and calmly, deep in sleep. His features no longer torn with cramp, his face looked almost relaxed.

As I sat on the edge of the bed half-relieved and half-shocked, I recalled that I had dreamt a most wonderful dream. I had seen Timmy laughing and happy in the water swimming with dolphins, a completely healthy child, with clear wide happy eyes, full of fun and happiness. At that time I had no idea how much this dream was about to influence and change my life.

Friends

Since that dreadful day of my son's accident, our lives changed completely. Nothing which seemed important yesterday remained of any consequence. From one second to the other our little family became disorientated.

Up to this fateful day our lives were filled with activities, exciting events and sometimes ,one could have said, glamor. Because of our professional surroundings and the long established friendships formed over many years, my husband and I found ourselves in the happy position of being surrounded most of the time by illustrious company. So often we had guests at home and I felt particularly happy in the role of the 'perfect hostess'. Our parties were famous — my home-made dishes almost world-famous and to prepare a menu of several courses for eight or ten or more persons was, for me, more of a pleasure than stress, and the compliments of my guests made it all the more worthwhile.

With the same ease I had borne my children, and as a mother, my life was filled. Especialy having two wonderful children, I was at the top of feminine joy and achievement.

To keep my independence after I was married I had formed, for security, an agency for sport sponsoring and event marketing. This was not only for glory, but also to follow the call, and armed with a desk, a phone and a typewriter as my office, I 'rolled up my sleeves' and set off on another professional path.

In the meantime all was not well with my marriage, it had began to crumble at the edges. Already during the course of my second pregnancy we had bad arguments which resulted in pre-natal and 'premature birth problems', so that I decided on a trial separation.

To be honest I did not really wish to separate from my husband at this time but felt that I had to do something which would shake and wake him up — make him realize how much I really needed him. I felt 'left out in the rain' and I missed the romantic side of happy pregnancy in harmony with my partner. This interlude brought about no change, only the misunderstanding of my entire family and I found out that the times when pregnant women had been treated with care and gentleness were long gone.

Sometimes today I long to experience a pregnancy with a partner who is 'more pregnant' than me, someone who takes over the worries and packs me in cotton-wool, who is able to cover over the changes in mood in a blanket of good humor and understanding.

Therefore in the light of day our marriage was not without its problems. But in spite of the daily battles I was still certain that this was the only man I had ever wanted to marry. I loved him. I loved him deeply and honestly. His body had never lost its fascination for me. If I was separated from him, I could not sleep well. I loved his smell, loved his gestures and loved his disarming smile. He was my husband and I wished for nothing more than that he should react differently and more positively to our arguments, and I wished for the patience that I did not possess. I wished for the diplomacy which was needed to make my 'six-foot' child grow into an adult man. I wished also for the presence of mind of a fully fledged woman to keep her mouth shut here and there.

For all of this I did not bring a lot of knowledge from my school of life, and so it was that almost daily I got my 'broom out of the closet' and in the course of the arguments 'flew off around the lamp' and was, even then, surprised that, after my landing, not everything had been sorted out.

Almost nothing was sorted out in our marriage. Regardless of what I asked of my husband he promptly forgot it. If there was something to be done, certainly he forgot to do it. Incidentally young fathers who care for their troubled babies at night must be the idea of TV producers! My husband played with the children, but only when he had an audience. Under these circumstances it was not easy to read in magazines about the new generation of fathers! In spite of all this my husband had the potential to be a really good father. He had no problem changing diapers and it was, at times, wonderful to see how he got on with the children when he actually applied himself. And both children loved him with all their hearts. When his father came home Timmy was always rosy-cheeked for sheer joy, and he did everything possible to gain his father's attention.

At the age of only four weeks Kira already started to try to flirt with her father. Everything could have been so perfect if only I could have stopped reminding him constantly that the role of father and husband demanded more than he was prepared to give. Perhaps all would have gone well had I had the patience to wait a few years in the hope that he would 'see the light' for himself.

So I feel inner peace that at the time of Timmy's accident we were together. I am pretty sure that if there had been the slightest suspicion that one of us had the chance to give the other any responsibility for the accident, with deadly certainty we would have destroyed one another.

So Timmy's accident was everybody's and nobody's fault. It was a collective guilt. Twenty-two adults and four children were with him when he disappeared. His closest relations were near to him, his uncle and great uncle the brightest stars in his scallywag life. All his partners for playing, joking and doing all those silly things, all our nearest and dearest friends, the family and especially his beloved grandmother, in whose presence all others faded from sight. And there he had been, next to my mother before suddenly he disappeared. It can only have been a matter of seconds before someone realized that he was missing.

All the people who were at Kira's baptism must surely still have to fight with the memories of what had happened. Immediately following the accident they came almost daily, not wanting to be alone, and to discuss and speculate and somehow together come to terms with the horrifying experience. As the immediate shock of the tragedy began to subside and no miracle happened, we suddenly found ourselves to be alone completely.

But for us the tragedy continued. I was certain that this accident would get my husband and me closer together again. I tried to see it as a sign of destiny that we should continue our way along life's path together. Therefore it was even more distressing for me to discover that my husband did not seem to even try to share this point of view.

He did not have the urge or the need to visit Timmy and me at the hospital, apart from the previously planned times. Nor did it occur to him to pack our little daughter in the car and bring her to see me, even if only for a few minutes. Rarely he watched at Timmy's bedside; when I arrived late because I was caught in a traffic jam or something else, he simply got mad at me. Our arguments increased in intensity and I could not understand why this father did not make more use of the key which he obviously had to his son.

I could hardly bear the despair over Timmy's condition and began to blame my husband for, in my eyes, all his failings. I wished with all my being that we could have shared the pain and cried together and then possibly have found strength in one another which we so desperately needed in order to survive.

Within our circle of friends odd things began to happen. Those whom I thought would always be there for me, for us, could not cope with the situation and so no longer found themselves strong enough to continue walking together with us. Others whom I had thought of as mere acquaintances, of no great depth, suddenly showed the energy and ability to give us courage.

At this time all, except us, continued with their normal lives. I noted this. It didn't bother me one way or the other. At that time I could not do anything for or against it. I found myself in a complete vacuum. At this point I was, most certainly, not a good partner for shallow conversation. With a large amount of disinterest and absolutely no degree of understanding I reacted to the phrases I heard such as, 'We just don't know how to help you'.

Of course it was difficult to reach me, but did I have to excuse myself for that? It made me really sick to see the phlegmatic reaction of some people. It became clear to me that I had made some severe mistakes in the characteristics of some of my so-called friends — I had obviously seen qualities which, in fact, they simply did not possess. As for some of the tips and advice I received, even from within my own family, I could not have given a damn.

I really believe that some 'old friends' of former times should be ashamed for the way they had behaved. Looking back it is surprising to note that in the place of the old friends, new ones suddenly appeared. If I would look today at a photo of my collective friends, those who I have known for an age, half my lifetime, are few and far between. People, who at the time of Timmy's accident I hardly knew or did not know at all, are now some of my closest friends and I feel as if I have known them my whole life. These people are at my side through conviction, to make me go on, to give me help when I am in need and of course to criticize when it is necessary — to prevent me from giving up when I feel that it's all too much. For the very first time in my life I now can be sure that I can rely on my friends.

The first in this line is Michael. We were business friends and at the weekend prior to Kira's baptism had realized our first major project together. He is the absolute professional, a gentleman of the old school with whom I would have sealed each deal with a handshake. A friend of my childhood days whom I had asked for advice on a new project of mine introduced us. When I mentioned that I did not know a 'Mr L.' the old fox was astonished. 'What! You want do business in this branch and don't know "Mr L."!' And so my friend arranged a meeting with this all-so-important 'Mr L'.

We were immediately sympathetic to one another, spoke the same language in terms of professionalism and had the same concepts and opinions regarding various projects. It was wonderful for me to have found such a valuable partner.

I had never viewed the branch in which I worked with my agency with great esteem. Although I enjoyed the work and the challenge of new projects, and to taking part in little intrigues of the business, now and again to watch how many of the actors playing their parts disregarded the value of Honesty, Openness, Loyalty and Honor. I assume that some of them would have been incapable of even spelling these words!!

But Michael was the exception that proved the rule in this business. A gentleman.

When I found myself on the Intensive Care Unit at the Hospital, with my child in a coma, I had to re-organize my life. At this time I was quite certain that my husband would be best helped in finding his role in this scenario by returning to work. I spent most of my time with Timmy anyway and it made me just nervous to argue about who had to do what.

When, on the first night he was due to stay with Timmy, and his major concern was 'Where am I supposed to sleep?', and he left my child in the care of the night-sister, the point was reached for me where I decided to relieve him of any responsibility at all. Then one Sunday afternoon he set his priorities by leaving a very anxious Timmy alone while he watched Formula 1 racing on TV in our rented room in the nursing sister's home. From this time on, I no longer put any value on his presence and preferred to continue alone.

In order to maintain contact with the outside world, with my family and with my daughter, all I needed was a cellphone.

Certainly there may have been other ways to quickly get a phone, but on the spur of the moment I called Michael, told him what had happened, and asked if he could get me a hire phone as quickly as possible, as I had no time to do this myself. He was sad to hear what had happened and promised to take things into his own hands immediately. At midnight on the same day he appeared in the clinic with his girlfriend, as if it was the most natural thing in the world to do a business partner a favor. I was deeply moved.

In the time following, my true and faithful friend never forgot, at least twice a week, to enquire about Timmy's state of health.

These conversations were balsam for my damaged soul, and when speaking with Michael, whom I still addressed formally, with my half-dead child in my arms, I felt that he was able to paint a very small glimmer of light for us on the horizon. We became a 'communion of souls' on the phone.

In a short period of time Michael became the anchor of my ship, which found itself in perpetual seas of torment. He was always there for me, for us, when I needed a friend. And so I asked him to help with some business matter or to take care of my broken down car. My husband and he became friends, especially through their common interest in cars. I was pleased that they both got along well and hoped instantly that some of Michael's fine and sensitive soul would rub-off on my husband.

Michael knew that behind my exaggerated gestures and bull-headedness against destiny lay my underlying despair. He never asked me 'How are you?' — he just knew that this question was unnecessary. The deep gentleness with which he looked at Timmy moved my heart for he, too, was touched by the state of my loved one. He knew instinctively when he was needed or when it was time to take his leave. Discreetly and without any desire for praise he was there. He taught me how to cry again and to transpose this relief into an iron will; he listened when I had the need to talk and tried to distract me at times of distress when I no longer wanted to live. He remained silent at the times when there was nothing to say. But he was always there for Timmy, for Kira and for me. Without him there would be no story to tell today, no book to write and no organization called *dolphin aid*.

For it was he who prevented me from ever giving up and to fight the urge to make an end of this life for Timmy and me.

Therapy — What is it?

Up until my son's accident a person who needed therapy was, for me, either mentally ill or a drug addict. Suddenly, from one day to the next, we were confronted with the most varied forms of therapy and forced to come to terms with them — things of which we had never even heard.

Then something began, which from my viewpoint was the most difficult task on the road to Timmy's recovery — the decision to choose which form of therapy would be the best for him, the most important, the most suited and that which would bring him the most help. We waited in vain for a reply from someone as to which therapy helped the most or was the most successful for a given child in a given situation. Already staff at the Intensive Care Ward at the Remscheid Clinic had began the sometimes fruitless search for the right way to bring my son back to a life of dignity and grace.

The first form of therapy prescribed for Timmy was the so-called Vojta Method. Professionals are at odds amongst themselves as to the value of this rehabilitational method. As Timmy's mother I had, from the very beginning, an aversion to this method because of the pain it caused Timmy.

Up until the time of the accident my son was a laughing and happy child. If he hurt himself I could easily soothe him in that I played the clown, kissed away the little injuries. He knew no hurt, no force and no pain.

How terrible it must have been for him, the first experience in his new shocking state, to undergo pain, moreover, to see me at his side letting it happen. Up to this point I had never imagined that anyone could cause my child pain in my presence — and how exactly was that supposed to help? I wanted to shout at the therapist, 'Get out. You're mad — stop hurting my child', but I was not able to at this moment because I was in a state of lethargy, carried forward by the hope that the people caring for my son were richer in experience and knew better than me what was good for him.

The first really positive and most important inspiration in my search for the right direction was in a book, written with much feeling, for which I thank the author Wolfgang Lechner with all my heart. In *Laugh Again Little Raphael* the father tells the story of his son, following a drowning accident. He writes of the unusual methods used by therapist Meike Weitemeier. His mention of her name made it possble for me to make a contact. For months I only knew Mrs Weitemeier from her very pleasant telephone voice. She was the person, who even a long time before she saw Timmy, set in motion the necessary activities and laid out the path.

During our first conversation on the phone I learnt that she was almost sixty years old. It was unbelievable, her voice was filled with energy, and dedication and *elan*. She could easily have been only 25 years old. She had a great wealth of experience and I would, with great respect, call her the Grand Dame of the German Physiotherapists.

With patience she heard Timmy's story and asked important questions at the relevant times. In spite of almost forty years experience she was really moved and her compassion really helped me and did me good. As I told her of the method of therapy they were using with Timmy at present she replied, 'Oh my god!!'. Thankful for this professional support, I set about putting an end to the Vojta Torture.

'Persuade this child to swallow', she said. 'You should do nothing else but encourage him to swallow. Give him as little as possible by drip and start drop-by-drop, using a syringe. The child must swallow. A child who cannot swallow cannot learn again to speak. Those who have no control over the mouth have no sense of balance. Fight off the doctors who want to introduce a line to the stomach through the abdominal wall, he would never again develop the feeling of hunger — do not allow them to do this! It will be a long and painful journey; there will be many times when you want to give in but persevere and start right away. Listen to me Mrs Kuhnert, Timmy must swallow.' Never was a call, an order, so penetrating. I was almost happy at last to have some clear directive and to have an aim with a positive goal.

With quite unknown strength I encouraged Timmy to begin swallowing again. At night I still fed him with calorie-rich foods by drip in order that he should lose no more weight, or at least retain his weight, but in the daytime I experimented with various nutritious appetizing fillings with the syringe. After about four months intensive training it was possible to feed Timmy, very slowly, minute portions with a spoon. It is interesting to note that in the medical release notes from one of the many clinics where Timmy was treated they wrote, under remarks, 'Improvements — We managed to persuade the patient to eat from a spoon'. I don't think I can find the words to say what I think about that!! — and I couldn't print it anyway!

By the end of 1994 Timmy was in such state that we could risk taking him to Mrs Weidemeier in Hamburg. Her slender and youthful person fully confirmed the impression which I had of her from the phone. With endless patience and with an astonishing willingness she gave herself completely over to Timmy and began with her work.

My son was still 'as stiff as a plank' as soon as he left my arms.

His eyes were filled with pain and an out-of-this-world look and at the same time filled with nothing — just emptiness. His limbs had started to distort. He moved his head in brutal movements into the neck, he bored into whatever he was laid upon so badly that after a few weeks the back of his head was bare, like a monk's tonsure. The rest of his hair became matted. His ribs and chest were extremely forced forward so that his back was equally concave. After only two minutes fight with the bedclothes, he had wounds on his elbows. His condition was pitiful and for that reason I could not even be really happy that he could swallow again. The dark and unseen forces which ruled Timmy's body and used him for their devices remained too strong.

How often did I think at that time 'If that's what life is, then we both don't want it', neither myself nor him. I caught myself in the moments of deepest anguish thinking about ending this pain for us both and yet in the same second felt shame for having entertained such thoughts.

Doctors, healers and 'quacks'

When I think back over the past it seems to me as if the birth of my two children is much closer in time than Timmy's accident and the terrible time which followed. This self-defense mechanism is a great gift. I don't think that anyone could survive such a severe stroke of fate without the blessing of forgetfulness. The ghastly pictures have not vanished from my memory, they recur again and again, even when I really wish that I could forget them. They fade a little with time, at least in daily life, and then make room despite the constant pain, for positive experiences.

In the course of time I have developed my own philosophy for the treatment of my son. Anything which does not hurt or damage him could, in theory, possibly help him to become a happy child again.

If we don't try something we will never know whether it may have helped. So, on our search for the solution to our problems, we have often walked strange paths.

When I think back I always followed, however stupid it might sound, an inner voice. I have such a powerful and strong bond with my son that I can interpret his signals as to whether a particular therapy should be stopped and another method tried.

Until today we have often gone fruitless and useless ways, and to do this, have undertaken expensive journeys. We have visited healers who were only people who called themselves healers and nothing else, and we have followed even the smallest glimmer of hope if we thought it may lead in the direction of recovery. And I am pleased that it was so, and that we took these ways, even when one or the other excursion only served to ruin my nerves even further. There is no doubt in my mind that I ever left untried a possibility of healing help.

At some stage my aunt, who lives in Mallorca, rang me. She had spoken about Tim with a dear friend of mine, the abbot of the monastery at Randa. He had told her that he knew of a Mallorquin doctor who treated brain damaged children, with great success, with acupuncture. She had studied with a specialist for acupuncture in Rome and wanted to come with her teacher to Germany in order to treat Tim. They both felt certain that they could help him.

I was euphoric and thankful for this offer of help and that my aunt had set all the wheels in motion already for the visit of the two doctors.

Following two days of observation the professor recommended us to come to Rome with Tim for at least three weeks so that he could continue the treatment. Tim was not the first little coma patient that he had treated, he said, but made it clear that it was of absolute importance to have the patient under observation for a specific period of time. He assured us that within six months Tim would return to full health. Who would not have, in the light of these promises, immediately packed their bags?

When I think of the circumstances of this journey it still makes me sick, and I must admit that I took Timmy to Rome under almost impossible conditions. To be truthful, at that time he was not really fit to travel. The whole story was to develop into a torture of unimaginable dimensions which drove all of those taking part to the brink of despair. Together with my mother-in-law who had travelled with us for support, we lived together in a large suite in a Roman hotel. Daily, Tim was treated by the professor. It was necessary to cross this huge city by taxi, in the rush-hour, with my spasm-ridden child in my arms and my nerves frayed. This would have been enough to give anyone the ultimate breakdown! But even worse than this — and hard to believe as it is — was that Tim reacted to the treatment with great agitation. From one second to the other he developed a high fever and his condition was serious. He had not only not improved — quite the reverse, his condition was to a great degree worse. We had spent a lot of money on the journey and the treatment, money which was not even ours — and on top of this we were robbed of one further hope.

Kira could just about crawl at this time and it was only due to her natural good nature that she was not branded by our disappointment and black mood. Even though today I know that this expedition of hope proved to have been a fool's journey, I don't regret that we did it. So at least I never have to think 'if only you'd gone to Rome'.

Naturally our friends and relations had stores of new tips for us. One time my mother, who is usually not impressed by the esoteric movement, saw in a newspaper an article about a so-called 'healer'. So one gloomy Wednesday afternoon we found ourselves in Frankfurt, in the overfilled practice of this man who was surrounded by sacred pictures and figures. After one glance at Timmy he reached the diagnosis — 'That will be 100 Bucks!', and said we should come back the following week! Let me tell you we didn't and ticked off another experience!

All these sobering episodes have not stopped my persistent search. Even when the methods have been strange, I sought further ways which could possibly help to make life worth living again for Timmy. And in the end we have found them!

It's a matter of fact that the German law in respect of 'Natural Healing' forbids me to name any of these extraordinary people who in fact did not cure Timmy, but were of immense help when he had problems with pneumonia, or in the fight against his pains or other minor sicknesses. These people gave not only Timmy, but also me, a little of the energy which I needed to continue my fight.

I even met one lady 'healer' who treated dogs, cats and even horses successfully. I think that any form of delusion in the mind's eye is not present with these patients! When this lovely lady treated Tim, and I held, at the same time, his hand or foot, even I was relaxed. I could have fallen asleep on my feet, and after a short period of time felt as if I could have torn out trees!

I remember with affection a story which occurred following my appearance in a popular TV show. About two weeks after the show I spoke to one of the producers, and he told me that he had received a very strange letter from some odd figure who wanted to treat Timmy. And he could not make up his mind whether to send me the letter or not. 'Are you mad', I shouted through the phone. 'Are you kidding me, you must be crazy? Someone wants to help my son, and you don't know if you should send me the letter?' The producer murmured 'He's only after money, and probably only wants to get on TV'.

'Well', I replied, 'if he can do anything to return Timmy to his normal state he certainly deserves media interest, and all the money in the world'. And so with this 'therapist' we got to know a new friend who travelled with us quite a way on our further journey. He, too, could not achieve any spectacular results but through his treatments was able to give my son, in his critical condition, the strength he needed. And so for that reason it was good that he was with us.

On the other hand I get really angry when I think of some of the doctors who treated Timmy. Recently I said to a very pleasant doctor 'My son, my daughter and I have managed to get this far, even though we were in medical care. Yes, you have understood properly — even though we were in medical care.' If *dolphin aid* didn't exist and if each day had a further twelve hours I would start another organization and that would be dedicated to the widening of understanding of German doctors at least!!!!

I really ask myself sometimes if having studied medicine gives someone the automatic right to act as an advisor on life or as a prophet, and to deliver mostly unasked for prophecies which not only destroy the future of a 'special needs' child, but also the future of entire families, not to mention the mental and physical state of the mothers!

Therefore I want to ask the question, using the example of my son, what dreadful state would he be in today if I had ever blindly listened to and believed all that the 'Gods in White' had told me?

I was told that Timmy should not have learnt to swallow again — but he swallows! Most doctors wanted to introduce a P.E.G., a tube into the stomach through the abdominal wall, just to make things easier.

He couldn't be expected to gain weight — but he has! He gained weight proportionate to his growth and at one time even had to be put on a diet because he had a few pounds too many! I was even told by one therapist that if he was not so fat he could already sit up by himself! And I remember clearly this so important university professor telling me, 'These children do not gain weight'. I replied, 'This child's name is Tim, this child is my son and for the rest we shall see'.

Strictly speaking he shouldn't be able to sit, just to lie, without any control over his head. Then Professor Brucker from the University of Miami gave us hope last autumn, that we may get Timmy on his own two feet, because he can already sit unsupported on my lap.

One professor told me that he, Tim, was not able even to recognize that I was his mother. A joke? But the truth is that Timmy can tell exactly who comes or goes, whom he likes or dislikes, who is important to him and to use Kira's words is 'one of our people'.

He shouldn't be able to hear. But the fact is that my son loves classical music; his favorites are Mozart and Bach. He gets upset if you disturb him during an interesting audio book. If his grandmother calls before he can even see her, his whole face lights up. Oh yes, he likes using the phone and gets quite cross if we speak with friends and relations and forget to give him the phone. And this 'dumb child' also understands every single word in English, which was proved by readings from a computer in the University of Miami School of Medicine.

He should not be able to see. To be truthful this is the only sense which is not yet fully restored. But that is why it is that much more wonderful when his bright blue eyes, with the depths of the sea, look into mine. That proves to me that at least he can see in intervals, but that it is still too tiring for him to digest inwardly all that he has seen.

A further list of the abilities which Timmy was 'never to possess again' — but has — would go on and on and no doctor can ever imagine the indescribable happiness when out of the time before the accident a cheeky grin, which we thought had been lost forever, appears on his face.

Needless to say Timmy is far away from being able to lead a normal, not to mention an independent, life. But he is a member of our family and we all do our utmost to give him a normal environment.

It takes a lot of energy, but it's possible. It's all built up like pieces of a puzzle — for instance the visits for an hour or two to the kindergarten, through a very wise decision made possible by a man from the town authorities and a very involved kindergarten-principal. After all the stress of therapy sessions and visits to various doctors it's a place he can let himself go and he truly enjoys the company of his healthy little friends. But before all this was possible, somebody had to ask for it.

I would love to shout out my message to all parents who find themselves in a seemingly hopeless situation with a 'special needs' child. 'Don't let anyone rob you of the natural feeling you have for your child. Listen to your inner voice, and decide for yourself what is right and important for your child. Force the doctors to listen to your point of view and your opinion and to take your anxieties seriously.' It is only committed parents who can give the sad lives of their 'special needs' children new meaning.

The time is ripe for change and I would go so far as to say that in my estimation about 40% of the handicapped children and young adults who are being kept in homes or hospitals at present could, with the help of better rehabilitation, lead at least a happy and independent life instead of just being kept fed, warm and dry in some institution.

Neither can I agree to the phrase 'One has to accept one's fate' or the one about 'You'll just have to come to terms with it'.

I just cannot hear this any more. I know of no example where the pure acceptance of destiny has led to any positive changes in life.

Love, thinking positively, keeping the family together, good friends, courage and laughing, even when at times these are the most difficult things to do, they are the base from which you can take on the fate which has been dealt to you. How much more important is it to transmit these principles epecially to children who rely upon the help of others.

Therefore I have a problem with the word 'handicapped'. What does it mean — 'handicapped'? Who handicaps whom and through what? The word itself seems so final, stupid — cripple — end — finished. But no-one asks how stupid and mentally handicapped some of the so-called healthy are, because they are not able to adjust themselves to the handicaps which others may have. I wish no-one a 'special needs' child and there again there are moments when I wish that, just for a fraction of a second, I could observe all the 'medical experts' who have laughed or belittled my efforts, dealing with such a situation. It's for sure that their forecasts and diagnoses would freeze on their lips and we, the mothers of 'special needs' children, would possibly meet them again in the most unlikely locations of this world as they, too, sought to do everything for their child.

Our family grows: Timmy's care team

After the tragic accident it took a very long time before I could accept that the care of a traumatized child like Timmy required the assistance of professionals.

Fifteen months after the accident I still had found no-one whom I would have trusted to assist in the care of my child with all the loving care and gentleness that he deserved and, in his dependence, so desperately needed. I must however accept the criticism that my search hadn't been very earnest, and that obviously I did not want to give anything up. In the end I had to accept that it was only possible to take proper care of my son and at the same time to give Kira the attention and support, bearing in mind that she had all the right in the world to experience and enjoy the most happy childhood possible under these circumstances. I needed help so I not only invited a nurse to an introductory meeting, I actually employed someone. It was about time!

At the beginning this also seemed to be a financial impossibility for me, but with the help of the manager of our medical insurance company we received the assurance that the costs for a nurse would be met by the company.

However, I have to admit that in the matter of nursing services I had already burnt my fingers, and as an example let me just mention that the last nurse who came to us for a trial of a few days tried to steal my husband's car. It was sheer luck that he took the keys of a car which was no longer in our possession.

Most of the people who came for an interview, I could tell after a couple of sentences, were not suitable candidates. They asked the wrong questions, did not appear to be flexible in any way or were simply looking for a job, not for responsibility.

Timmy's condition definitely required specific qualifications which I was not able to see in the majority of applicants. In the end remained the feelings of a mother. I wouldn't even trust them enough to put my child into their arms.

And so for a further year and a half I continued with my tightrope act between night-watch duty, children's room, kitchen, office, clinic, therapy and all other appointments, only with the help of our Philippine maid.

I will never forget when she told me, one time, right after Timmy's first return from a hospital, that her brother had had the same diagnosis as Timmy and that she had cared for and nursed him. I almost exploded — I thought quite simply that she had misunderstood exactly what the situation was here. But I had done her an injustice. It was really true. At the age of 9 her brother had a drowning accident in Bulacan in the Philippines and his condition, after the misfortune was, as she said, almost the same as Timmy's. She had nursed him, and she told me that from the accident there remained, in the end, only a spastic disability in the right hand. She said to me over and over again, 'Believe me Mrs Kuhnert, my brother was like that'.

So Lerma became a source of energy and a wandering memorial to trust faith and hope. She grew far above herself — small and delicate as she was, she carried Timmy everywhere through the house, for it was still not possible, even for a second to not be in physical contact with him, otherwise he would have stopped breathing immediately. She sang to him and cared for him with a gentle sensitivity, a mixture of intuition and love. Naturally she had no medical training and so I could never leave her alone with all the responsibility. But at last I had a partner who enabled me to spend time with my daughter and also to be able to take a deep breath, here and there.

And so our little circle closed — Timmy accepted my husband, Lerma and me as a trio. We, the women, developed previously unknown talents, with the little 'Kackalafutzi' in our arms; to make a cup of tea, do the housework, make the important telephone calls and so on.

Now and then I have dressed myself and put on my make up with him still in my arms, feeling as if I was a circus act, but at least when I looked in the mirror then I did not have the permanent feeling that I was half dead — although I actually looked dreadful.

Timmy's grandparents felt most unhappy in their helplessness for even in their arms he found no peace. He was most rigorous on this point, to be carried and guided through this world, he accepted only Papi, Mami and Lerma and that was it! So how in the world could I find someone in this situation who would be a suitable strengthening of our team? In the meantime Lerma had become part of the family and was on her feet up to 16 hours a day for us, and that at least six days a week. In this time our household help, without whose help I would never have managed either to maintain my strength, let alone my nerves, became my closest ally.

But nevertheless it was crystal-clear that I must make a decision.

On one of his many business trips abroad my husband had got into conversation with an English colleague and spoken about my situation and my fears. He told my husband that nurses from Great Britain were not only extremely well qualified and well trained but were instilled with a natural gift of combining nursing with care. We decided therefore to advertise the position of nurse in England and to bring a British nurse, who would live with us and be a strengthening partner for Timmy, to Germany.

That was how Jaqui came to us.

On the very first evening at the meal table I had the feeling that I was sitting opposite, and chatting with, an old friend. We had already talked through all the major points of our working together and I was relieved to discover how much we had in common, including our sense of humor.

Jaqui Nicholl was an enrichment to our team. Her natural and uncomplicated manner made the loss of our intimate private atmosphere less drastic. Her little quirks, which we all have, were overlooked exactly as those of other members of the family. She was a real 'sleepy-head' in the mornings and so if possible I tried not to organize anything for her before 10 in the morning! Nevertheless there were times when I went off the deep-end, shouting through the house 'Nicholl! — I'm not your servant!'.

Although she was most competent when it came to dealing with medicines, disinfection and all other things connected with medical care, in all other areas I can say, without malice, that she was a little crazy. The shock I got when I went up to the attic apartment, where she had made her home in the house, was like a hammer. It was unbelievable that someone who was otherwise a cultivated person could live in a place that looked as if it had been hit by a bombshell. But Jaqui managed to and felt quite happy.

It didn't really matter how this jovial Irish girl managed her private life because she was a fantastic nurse, wonderful and gentle companion for Timmy. In Kira's life she played a major role, was a valued playmate and one of her closest allies.

For a whole year, a very difficult year, Jaqui was with us. My marriage had finally broken down, Timmy had to face surgery twice, he had also had his first Dolphin Human Therapy and I was constantly concerned about Kira's further development, that she should not be damaged in any way by the situation. After this year we had to say goodbye to this 'crazy Irish nurse' who had been for all three of us like a sheltering port in a storm. It was a very sad parting, I cried my eyes out because Jaqui had become a great and close friend whom I will never forget. She had gone through thick and thin with me, we had laughed and cried together many times. That had given us both a great deal, but I could not live her life nor she could live mine.

When Jaqui left, it was also a valuable lesson for the children — saying goodbye is another part of a relationship however hard that may be. Loving someone is also being able to let them go.

And so she flew off back to Ireland, to her friend Ian, to get married and to start a family of her own — with one great wish in her heart, to have a daughter like her little 'princess', like Kira.

Two years later Cara was born. We have all got to know this little lady and we are all very happy when Jaqui comes to visit us and chats with the children in English — she still doesn't speak more than three words of German! But for this reason the foundation stone was laid that Kira quite simply grew up bilingual and that Timmy too understands both English and German — all quite naturally. For a long period of time we spoke only English at home and often wondered in which language Timmy would say his first word, when he learnt to speak again.

The loss of Jaqui as my 'co-pilot' was difficult to cope with and it was to be another six months before I found a suitable replacement for her.

Along with Piroschka Kaiser the third language entered our home and this time it was Hungarian. At the beginning understanding one another was not without its problems, it was almost impossible! She too spoke more or less no German, my Hungarian was even worse. This situation caused a few uproars in the house and when I asked 'Did you understand me?' she would blithely answer '*Ja, ja*' although she had not the slightest idea what I was talking about. The result was that I developed the skills of pantomime in order to make clear what the next step was in our daily routines.

Even today we often laugh about the fact that Piroschka, with a smile on her lips, could call me to my face a 'silly cow' in her own language, and I had not the slightest idea what she was saying!!

Hungarian still sounds strange to my ears. When Piroschka's mother, Magdolna, comes to visit us we understand one another very well although we each haven't the foggiest idea what the other is saying!

You could describe Piroschka's development like that of a butterfly. When she came to us she was a nice caterpillar, somewhat unsure because her lack of German. She had left Hungary for the first time in her life and was terribly homesick. Although we all tried our best to make her understand that she was part of the family, it took a long time before she really settled in.

She gave loving attention to the children even though there were problems with understanding and she quickly established a warm relationship with both of them. Kira put her to some hard tests to see whether she could really take a place like Jaqui has in her life.

At first I missed a jolliness in her character, and it was difficult to raise her enthusiasm for anything, but she gave all her energy over to the duties required of her regarding Timmy, and this from the heart.

In the meantime our Piroschka has become a beautiful butterfly. She speaks almost perfect German, in fact she has quite a talent for languages. She can manage well in English and even speaks a few words of Spanish.

Each day her professional skills increase and her personal development has produced a self-confident and very attractive lady.

If it goes on at this rate the day will come when someone asks 'Mrs Kuhnert, how long have you been working for Mrs Kaiser?'!!

Timmy has changed the lives of many people, and not one of these in any way negatively. Lerma, Jaqui and Piroschka all know deep in their hearts that this 'special little boy' has opened up for them new horizons and taught them to think in another way. In return for this gift they have accompanied us along the long and stony path towards a better future for Timmy. They have been valuable companions along the way for Kira and helped her to grow up to become a confident young lady. And I hope they know, all of them, that they have a very special place in my heart.

The first contact with Dolphin Human Therapy

In the middle of the night the phone rang. The operator asked me if I would accept the charges for a call from the USA, a Dr David Nathanson was on the line. At last!!!!

I was immediately wide-awake and overjoyed that I would speak to this man, for whom I had been searching for so long.

Dr Nathanson, the founder of Dolphin Human Therapy, is the first scientist to prove that children with many and varied handicaps learn up to ten times quicker when they work together with dolphins.

I was sure that this form of therapy could be the big chance for Timmy. However, because in the past, I had had so many pretty bad experiences and gone off on many fruitless journeys hope-filled, I first wanted to hear Dr Nathanson's opinion.

He took a great deal of time to discuss Timmy's situation with me, and recommended that for the first time I should fly alone to Miami and get a full picture of things for myself 'with my own eyes'.

Before committing Timmy to a ten hour flight in his sometimes dangerous medical condition I needed to be sure that the hopes and possibilities that I connected with the dolphins would warrant this pilgrimage.

Following this night-time call I was almost euphoric, and had a goal to go for, and felt that this could be the signal of a new possibility for Timmy.

Somehow it seemed natural to me that I should undertake this trip to Florida alone, for although I received support and advice from all sides especially from Timmy's rescuer, following the accident, I had always thought that I was, and felt myself to be, totally alone.

Nevertheless I felt relief when my husband, who either from lack of knowledge or because it was just easier, left it to me. When he, at least morally, supported my decisions, when he at least sometimes was physically present, I felt the loneliness deep inside of me was less present.

The nearer the date of my departure date came the more certain I was that this time I did not want the whole thing in my hands only. This time I didn't want to have the responsibility of solitary decisions, this time I didn't want to be the one to have the final and, most of the time, the only word.

Before I could discuss with my husband the possibility of going to Florida together, I had to organize an army of helpers for my children.

My mother agreed to take over the command in my absence on the condition that there were enough professional careers on hand. In the light of this she was prepared to take over the special duties in the field of kisses and hugs.

Barbara the physiotherapist wanted to stay overnight so that she would always be there for the necessary treatments at home. Lerma, our Philippine maid, was also willing to 'move in'. She had a valuable connection with Timmy and was, apart from myself, the only one who could continually feed him. Dr Mandl promised likewise to be available on call 24 hours a day and even gave me his private phone numbers. Christian, my assistant at the agency, wanted to set himself up in my office at home and be available as a chauffeur.

I committed the daily schedules to paper, wrote the important 'Marching Orders' down, started to cook like a maniac and prepared in advance the necessary daily medicines, for the exact time I would be away. I booked a second ticket to Miami.

I had finally compiled a list of all the emergency numbers, when I asked my husband if he could accompany me on the trip. I told him of my uncertainty and that I wished for nothing more deeply than that we should undertake this journey together in order to make the right decisions for Timmy. He seemed at least kind of relieved and promised to make this three-day trip possible. For the first time in ages he held me in his arms that night.

With a feeling I cannot fully describe — a feeling of fear that something could happen in my absence, and the excitement of the possibilities in Florida, which could be the key to open the door to a better quality of life for my son — I sat next to my husband in the plane.

My husband — how I had loved to say that word, and how hard it is to say it today. With this phrase 'My husband' everything was connected for me. Belonging together, warmth, love, our future, the present and also the past. My husband, the only man to whom I ever said 'Yes' with no reservations, with whom I had wanted to spend the rest of my life and from whom I have two wonderful children. My husband, the man I adored, and who was the purpose in my life. With his name everything for which the love of a woman stands was connected. Even now his name sounds so familiar, so near. All those little pet names I once had for him come into my mind — names which reflected my deep love but which I haven't spoken for years as desire faded.

Somewhere along the journey together we have lost one another and never found the way back again. Possibly because our lives became different. He was not able to find his way in the world of clinics, hospitals, dramas and anxieties.

Somehow it seems to me that he had never even tried to search for me and I did not have the understanding nor the indifference, to follow him after all that had happened, in his almost unchanged life-style.

For the first time in ages I looked at him quite consciously and was suddenly, 30,000 feet up in the air, more woman again, more than just the mother of a severely sick son and a little daughter. He's very attractive. I had always thought he was good-looking, a manly character.

I knew him so well. It felt good to see him from this perspective and it was as if I could feel the magic from the time when our love was young. I wished we could have started again and discovered one another anew.

New hope was born within me; hope that this journey would not only be a new start for Timmy but also for us. We were, at last, alone for the first time in ages.

On arrival at the hotel in Miami we found, waiting for us, a fax from Michael in which he wished us all the luck in the world. I could read between the lines and I knew that he understood the meaning I saw in this journey. That night in our hotel room I waited for a sign from my husband and hoped that he would take me in his arms; but he chose to hide his uncertainty behind the TV remote-control.

The following morning we set off very early. I had forgotten the disappointment of the previous night and tried to concentrate only on the reason we were here in Florida. And so I tried to enjoyed the drive to Key Largo, which lies about seventy miles south of Miami.

The fifth phone-call home confirmed that all was well at base, that Timmy's condition was stable, that Kira, in grandma's care, felt 'perfectly fine' and they tried to convince me that the kids did not miss me 'too much'. I felt in a good mood, almost relaxed and did not let myself be influenced by the usual less-than-euphoric, early morning mood of my husband. With every milestone we passed my expectations increased. I was so excited and curious about the animals and most of all about the therapy. How often had I questioned myself in the last few days as to what my expectations were. I didn't believe Dolphin Human Therapy to be a miracle-cure, but deep in my heart I did believe this could do just a great thing for Timmy.

After a drive of about an hour and a half we arrived at the therapy center Dolphins Plus where Dr Nathanson worked at that time.

The entrance was like a barn door in some southern European country and opened on to its own world. It was as if one had left a great piece of reality behind. The surrounding noises were gigantic. The welcoming calls of the dolphins mixed with the screams of the seagulls and other water fowl. And even though the noise was immense the whole place gave out an indescribable atmosphere of tranquillity.

Dr David Nathanson greeted us warmly. What we saw was a man who had nothing in common with the image which we were used to from German scientists and doctors. He was much more the genial grandfather type who possibly could spur on a horde of grandchildren to silly games and even bring laughter to the faces of their parents.

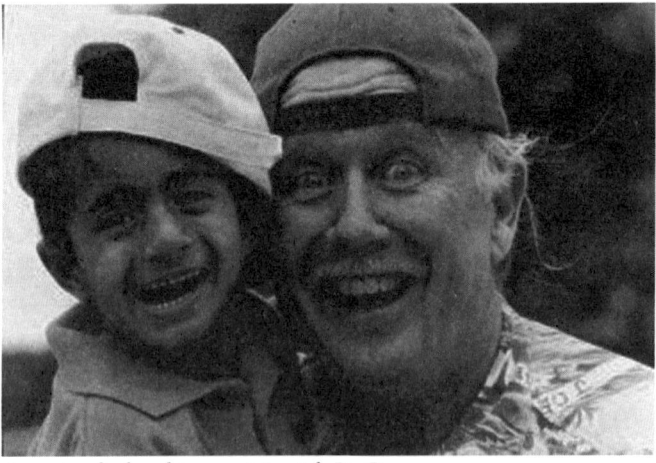

Learning by laughing: a visit with Dr Dave

His 'professional clothes' underlined this. Instead of the usual white coat, he had on shorts, a Hawaii shirt, tennis socks and sneakers.

As a crowning glory he had on his scholarly head a breathtaking cap which gave the impression that he had a dolphin growing out of his forehead, and whose tail fin, at the back of the good doctor's head, waved in co-ordination with his infectious laughter.

He had all the details of our previous conversations still in mind. There was no nurse in the background eagerly reading down from copious notes. His direct and precise questions could give the impression that he had occupied himself, in the meantime, solely with the interests of my son.

To my great surprise my husband spoke at length with Dr Nathanson, obviously pretending to be well-informed about Timmy's condition and it appeared that he at least had listened to my descriptions. Is this the same man for whose help in daily life I have often sought, to no avail?

Today I was in a good mood — and so I left him to do his thing.

Dr Nathanson explained to us the way the therapy ran. Today was an orienteering session which meant that first of all the patients make acquaintance with both the human and animal therapists.

The team around Dr Nathanson come from the most varied branches of rehabilitation. There are physiotherapists, psychologists, speech pathologists, occupational therapists and specialists in behavioral management. The location of the therapy is a natural creek set back and cut off from a waterway used by small boats. There are four docks from which the actual therapy is conducted.

Medicine balls, playthings with handles, exercise mats, symbol boards, color tables and rings are all there ready for use by the children — just as in any therapy practice. Using these utensils, an individual therapy program is created for each child.

Dr Dave introduced us proudly, almost with the air of a Father presenting his own children, to the key figures in this therapy: the dolphins Dingy, Squid, Fonzie, Alfons, LB, Kimbeth, Jeannie, Spunky and her baby Duke.

I am not only impressed by these extraordinary animals, I am moved and feel myself taken completely in by them. I could have just dived into the water, and let myself be carried by these animals, simply to swim with them, to imitate their movements and to experience the same ease with which they master the waters. Almost magnetically they draw me to them. I long to touch them and sink myself in the endless gentleness of their eyes.

A feeling of peace and warmth envelopes me. I am not, by nature, a contemplative or a balanced meditator, in fact it is the opposite. I usually need quite a distance from 'the now' to find peace with myself. In addition, water, by far, is not my element. And nevertheless I am drawn to the edge of the docks and feel an enormous desire to be part of this particular wet world and its inhabitants. For a second I forget everything, even Timmy and Kira, I am completely alone with my inner self and the dolphins, and for just one moment, which seems a little eternity, I step out of this world.

Dr Nathanson brought me out of this dream with a knowing smile.

The patients had arrived and, with the consent of the parents, he told us a little about each of the children and their various handicaps.

I couldn't really concentrate properly. I was watching a girl of about sixteen sitting paralyzed in her wheelchair. Her eyes seemed completely dead, and there was, mirrored within them, a well of sadness. Totally inactive she cowered in her terrible vehicle. She had a beautiful face, a slender and fine-limbed body which was numbed by sorrow. She'd had a motor accident which had left her with unspecific paralysis from the fifth vertebrae, so Dr Dave told me, but she was not a clear paraplegic case.

Donny the therapist carried her, with great care, onto the therapy platform, speaking to her the whole time. The girl gave the impression that she had fully distanced herself from her surroundings, as if to say 'Just leave me alone, no one can help me'. She worked at being totally shut-off. Even though she was much bigger, and her illness was in no way related to that of Timmy's, I strongly remembered this same apathy in my son.

Very carefully Donny brought her legs to the edge of the platform, so that her feet were dangling in the water. Out of nowhere Dolphin Dingy appeared before her and gently prodded her foot and then glided with the full length of his beautiful body past her, stroking her feet with his motion. As a reward dolphin trainer Lynn gave her strokes of acknowledgement and, of course, a fish.

Dingy seemed to take over the command herself and with heart-melting gestures tried to gain the attention of the girl. She sprayed her with water and 'chattered' constantly at her, she sprang before her, to dive again into the water so that she could plant another foot-kiss and a foot-prod. Did I suddenly see a smile? ... As if caught in the act the girl's face returned again to stone.

Without ever having spoken to this girl, I am sure that at the end of this twenty minute session, it must have done her good.

I had a long conversation with one of the lady therapists who had treated her own son. He was born with a heart problem. During the course of the first operation his heart had stopped beating. They had managed to revive him but he was left with brain damage.

His condition then seemed to be hopeless. The doctors advised her to come to terms with it, that her son would be, for the rest of his life, a severe nursing case. His condition following the operation seemed to me to be similar to Timmy's. 'And what is the state of things today', I ask her, naturally needing to know exactly. 'He has a slight problem in learning, but otherwise he has developed perfectly normally.' Almost hysterically I begin to laugh, I know now that I am in the right place for Timmy, and I tell her that I would probably be permanently in a state of hysteria if my son recovered from this tragedy with only slight learning problems.

With a heavy heart I take my leave on this first day and promise to come back the following day. On the return journey to Miami my husband and I hardly speak. Only after we call our parents to describe our impressions and what has happened do we speak with one another. It seems that we both have a feeling similar to happiness, especially as everything at home is OK.

We went for a long walk through Miami Beach that evening and later met, almost by chance, under the shower. For the first time in ages I fell asleep with some kind of a happy feeling. My dream was beginning to come true. Timmy would swim with the dolphins and he too would become happy again. Of that I was quite sure.

Our arrival in Key Largo the following day had something familiar about it, all the crew welcomed us as if we were old friends. On this morning I experienced the first little miracle of the Dolphin Therapy. The sad girl of the day before was being wheeled to the dock by her aunt. Upright in the wheelchair was a smiling, almost happy-looking young lady. I could hardly believe it.

Naturally I could not tell if she eventually learnt to move unaided. I would love to know her name, in order to tell her of the part she played in convincing me of the value of this therapy. I saw with my own eyes what the dolphins and the therapist achieved in the course of only just one day, giving back to this girl a piece of the quality of life, which is beyond price. And that for me is something truly fantastic. I looked towards my husband and our eyes met — we were in unison — Timmy must get here as soon as possible. Whatever the cost!!!

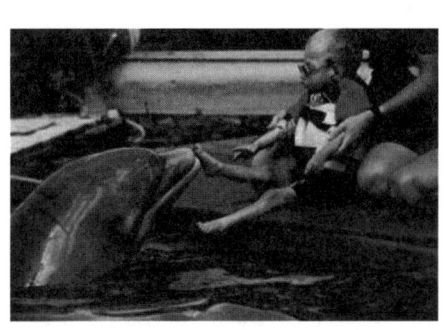

Dolphin Alphons during a therapy session

Dr Nathanson and his Team

Anyone meeting Dr David Nathanson for the first time, near to his therapy docks, would be first inclined to ask 'Where can I find Dr Nathanson?'. This is because nothing in his dress or his manner would lead you to think that this is the person who, to date, has helped several thousand children, from over fifty different countries, to take the step into a better Quality of Life with the assistance of Dolphin Human Therapy.

His working clothes nearly always consist of a pair of shorts, Hawaii shirt and sneakers. The muscular calves give some indication of his sporting past as a long distance runner and basketball player.

His face is freckled with the Florida sunshine, and often a little red.

The son of Scottish immigrants says himself that British, or rather Scottish, skin is not designed to be placed in the Florida sunshine!

Dr Dave, as he is called by everyone, was born on 15 May, 1945 in the astrological sign of Taurus. At three years of age little Dave could already read. During the course of his entire schooling he was always the youngest student in his class. Up until his fourteenth birthday he had only interested himself in Basketball, but then, according to reports, revised his ideas, and from that time forward gave 'girls' as his hobby.

At just sixteen years of age he registered at University. When I asked him why he had chosen the subjects of English Literature and Philosophy, he replied, with his usual cheeky grin, that those were the departments where the prettiest girls were. In order to finance his studies he accepted any job that was going, and these included truck-driver, factory worker, and whatever one could have imagined. He was fired from a warehouse job for fooling about the whole day. His father, a doctor of Russian descent, was not amused when young Dave decided to join the Civil Rights Movement, to fight for the voting rights of the black population in the Southern States. Even today Nathanson freely admits that he is still a friend of the 'underdogs'.

Following successful studies, he became a teacher. Being regarded as a child as highly talented, he began to teach gifted children. Parallel to this he studied at night for his Master of Science degree.

In an interview with the *People Magazine* he was later reported as saying that teaching highly talented children who received their gifts from nature was no 'big deal', but to teach a child who had never said a word in his life to speak, that really is a 'big deal'. Thereby the scientific assistant decided once again to return to University and began a study of Medicine. In 1973, at the age of 28, he became a fully qualified Professor at the Florida International University.

In the meantime Nathanson became, not only a husband and the father of two daughters, but also a

Doctor of Cognitive and Neuropsychology, and worked at the University of Minnesota principally on the connection between the brain and bodily functions. During this period of time he discovered that 'special needs' children have major problems of learning and developing in the areas of developing an attention span, and concentration. Following his observations that children especially love music, animals and water he came upon an adventurous idea — to work with the combination of handicapped children and dolphins.

Without further thought he drove to Fort Lauderdale, and spoke with the directors of Ocean World and presented his ideas. When he then asked 'Can you help me?' Dr Dave told me that he had expected a reply that recommended he have his sanity checked. But the reaction of the directors was completely different from what was expected!

'You can work with the dolphins up until 10.30 a.m. and after that we are open to the public as usual.'

And so, in 1978, the first pilot project, a study with 4 children, was established in Ocean World, Fort Lauderdale. The results were impressive. Dr David Nathanson found himself on the right path!

Before David Nathanson continued his studies at the Dolphin Research Center in the Florida Keys, there was a pause of six years. During this time he worked as a Forensic Psycholigist for the Justice Department in connection with cases connected with hardened criminals.

Finally, in 1988, the first detailed study was released with the results of scientific investigations at the Dolphin

Research Center, and published in the book *Clinical and Abnormal Psychology*.

Up until 1994 Dr Dave was only able to work with 'special needs' children and give them therapy two days a week, so the waiting list for Dolphin Human Therapy increased to a very long seven years! An impossible situation — and for this reason Nathanson asked Lloyd Borgus, the owner of Dolphins Plus, a unique dolphin facility in Key Largo, for help.

From this first request everything grew. In the course of time a friendship between these two extraordinary men developed. The result was that, in 1995, for the first time, a daily Dolphin Human Therapy program, in co-operation with Dolphins Plus in Key Largo, Florida, USA, began.

David Nathanson had achieved his goal. And as with many pioneers of new forms of therapy or new scientific practices, the people who swim against the current, trends and rules, it would often be questioned — is this man a genius, or is he quite simply mad? I am personally certain that history will prove the first to be correct.

Dr Dave's team is composed of professionals from many different branches.

They are all quite special personalities, who, together, master enormous tasks.

There is, for example, Marcia McMahon, a wonderful therapist, especially with autistic children. She is, as are her colleagues, purely and simply an idealist, for she is truly aware that she cannot become a wealthy woman from doing this job.

As a therapist Marcia is a marvelous mixture of the professional who also has the great talent of personal engagement. With extreme sensitivity, she knows what is right for her little patients.

She is a supporter of the classical behavioral theories, and is able to combine her knowledge of this subject with quite remarkable therapeutic intuition. Marcia has the ability to 'crack the hardest nuts' when it comes to difficult cases, and can reach the most stubborn or spoilt-child and the little princes like Timmy. She is able to awaken the will in them to work together in the therapy.

Each family who has had contact with Marcia has been able to return home with increased knowledge of their child. And the children miss her very much!

Dee Dee, whose real name is Diane Sandelin, is the co-ordinator for the volunteers from all over the world. She was a student of Dr Nathanson and so first came into contact with his work. For ten years the educationalist and swimming teacher for disabled children has been working together with Dr Dave. The 'senior therapist' in the team is a cheerful character with motherly instincts who arouses much confidence and trust — there are quite a few who have cried on her shoulder! Although over 50 you would never think so when you see her. When she speaks to the parents she knows exactly what she is talking about. Dee Dee is the mother of four, and her youngest daughter Lisa suffers from an extreme affliction of the spinal cord.

Christina Collins is the soul of the office of Dolphin Human Therapy in Key Largo. The exact description of her job is Director of Public Relations but this does not 'hit the nail on the head'. The half Austrian who also speaks a little German is really the 'Jack-of-all-Trades' when necessary. She translates during the treatments, works as an assistant to the therapists, she deals with communication and co-ordination — so then she communicates and co-ordinates, organizes and does lots of telephoning, she does hospitality and connects, arranges and, most of all, understands.

The rest of the team is supported in rotation, or as required by Speech, Occupational or Physio-therapists.

Dr Dave has composed a fantastic troop of people for 'his' children. They all work together during the therapy season from February until December, around the clock no matter whether it is Memorial Day, the 4th of July, St Patrick's Day or any other public holiday. And what is really an important matter for the success of this unique therapy is the happy, caring and cheerleading attitude of the entire Nathanson Crew. For families used to sorrow, this fact is a beautiful relief.

But what would the crew from Dolphin Human Therapy be without the real Dolphin People, the trainers — to put it in a nutshell, they would be in quite a mess.

The man who it is all about in this case is Rudolf. He is of German origin and, in 'the world of dolphins', one of the most respected experts.

Rudolf is an absolute phenomenon — not only for the animals but also for the people. His dolphins love him. He is the Alpha animal, he is the leader of their pack, the Boss, father, mother, friend and companion. He loves the animals as if they were his own family. He hardly ever takes a day off because he feels totally allied to his animals. They need his company and he needs theirs. In his contact with the other people — humans — it is another story.

Rudolf goes to a lot of trouble to make other people think that he is a grumpy, bad tempered, slightly eccentric person not inclined to conversation, just so that no-one scratches on his thick shell. He prefers to avoid chit-chat and, when he speaks, enjoys best a good argument.

In order to pass judgement on a person he first of all sends one of his dolphins.

When someone finds his opinions to be O.K., they can be lucky and find themselves as one of the selected persons who can get near to him. Then finally when one takes into account a few grumpy remarks, does not give up, and in the end wins the heart of Rudolf, one finds he is filled with integrity, reliable and the heartiest friend one could wish for. This side of his character is only exposed to the crew on most infrequent occasions. Meredith, who I adopted in mind and heart as my second daughter, Mary, Brigitte and Gereth could all write a book about his cursing and moody attacks. But nevertheless they show him all the greatest respect and also their affection. Each and every one of them knows that it is Rudolf who has made them what they are today, and that is excellent Dolphin Trainers, with the necessary sensitivity for the animals and the people. Teaching the ability to co-ordinate the dolphins, therapists and a handicapped child during a therapy session is most certainly the genius of Rudolf Jäckle.

And nobody has the slightest doubt about that!

All of those who strive, daily to bring a little light into the murky world of special needs children from all over the world are fantastic characters. One could talk about each and every one of them all day long.

They are one big family and, without exception, have all become my friends.

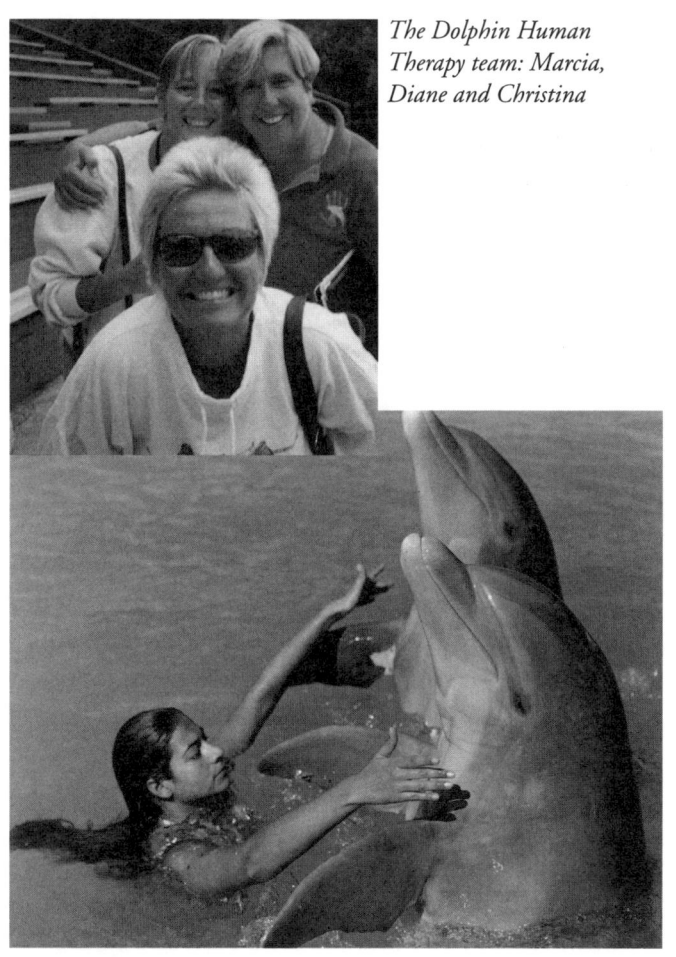

The Dolphin Human Therapy team: Marcia, Diane and Christina

Dolphin trainer Meredith and her beautiful animals

Timmy's first trip to the dolphins

Out of dreams the reality is born. Some ten months after the dream I had whilst I was sleeping on the field-bed in the University Hospital, where I had the wonderful vision of my son laughing and happy, I started the preparations for our first joint visit to Spunky, Duke, Dingy and the other dolphins.

During these preparations of adventurous proportions, much like the exodus of the Children of Israel from Egypt, I found myself constantly lost in day dreams, and asked myself how Timmy would react to the animals and the water. My impressions remain cloudy.

I wished so passionately for ... yes, what did I wish for exactly? I wished and hoped for a change, a clear signal for all to see, including those who treated Timmy as if he were just a piece of meat — someone who was not even worth considering as a puzzle or a mystery. I wished for a sign to be given to everyone, those to whom we ran and had begged for help, for those who hadn't even greeted my son before a medical examination, and those who, in retrospect, I am still completely sure wouldn't even have noticed if I hadn't brought my child for treatment.

I wished for a signal for those who didn't know his magical voice, and those who did not know how unbelievable it felt when he put his little arms around my neck — and for those who never bothered even to ask.

Of course I wished that these cramped arms could reach out again around my shoulders. I wished that his constant fists were once again relaxed and his open hands could stroke my face. I wished for a happy son who would recognize that it's well worth continuing living in this damned world, and who, in spite of his condition, is prepared to fight in order to become happy again.

Without doubt I had no exaggerated expectations of that which the dolphins could achieve for Timmy. I didn't expect him to suddenly get up and throw his, far too heavy, wheelchair into the ocean.

Even though every morning since the accident I wished that this nightmare would end, that Timmy would lie in his bed beaming at me and murmur something like 'Mami, Tinny awake', it was quite clear to me that he would never ever suddenly say 'So, Mami the fun is over — you did a good job, you weren't bad at all!'.

I wished for a positive change, however small that might be. And for that reason, following our return from Miami, in spite of the oppressive and strained atmosphere in our house, I fought not to lose hope.

It was a dreadful time. One of my husband's uncles had died, admittedly at a great age, but he left a great gap behind him. Tanti, his wife, was in total despair, for he had been her life and now she remained behind alone. I couldn't even attend the funeral because Timmy's condition gave too much cause for concern.

My Grandmother was ill with cancer of the throat. My beloved Grandma, the star of my childhood days, and the very first person I had told that I was expecting my first child. I remember clearly the day when she told me that 'something was not right with her'. She had absolutely no appetite and would vomit up even the smallest portion of food. I suggested that she immediately consult a doctor, and when she did not answer with the usual protests, I knew it must have been something serious. During the time I was packing the cases for America she was in a world between here and there and also floating between Intensive Care Unit and the regular nursing wards. Over and over again I suffered from a bad conscience. Could I go and leave her alone?

Every day I sat, for at least a few minutes, on her bed and spoke with her. Not knowing whether or not she could really understand me, I told her about the forthcoming trip. I explained to her how important this journey for Timmy was, how much I loved her and how much I needed her, that I found it unfair that she too had stopped speaking to me, that she couldn't leave me alone — and please, please get well very quickly.

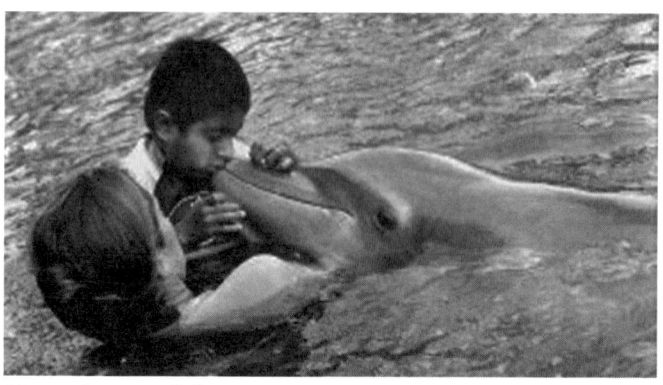

No words are needed ...

My mother gave me strength, washed my troubles away. She made it quite clear that it was perfectly in order for me to go to Florida for two weeks, and that in the meantime she would take especially good care of my beloved grandmother. And, for certain, I would be back for her 80th birthday.

And so came this Saturday in October 1995, as we, like a procession, set off. Timmy, Kira, my husband, Jaqui and myself, hopefully to find Timmy's chance of happiness in Florida, with 40 kg excess baggage and high hopes that weighed a great deal more.

Thanks to the kindness and care shown to us by my former colleagues, the check-in at the airport went without any problems. There were two extra seats reserved on board the aircraft, for Timmy's 'Journey of Hope.' This allowed enough space for us, our many pieces of hand baggage, space to stow all the things we needed by us in case of emergency: the oxygen, the suction pump, the medicines and also the special foods.

The other passengers on this flight probably imagined I was an immigrant, with my huge quantity of baggage.

To avoid such embarrassment, in the future, I usually used the Late Night Check In service of LTU airlines. Under the cloak of darkness I could check in my up to 25 pieces of luggage, without having to endure the sympathetic gaze of fellow travellers. There were always fragile pieces which had to be dragged off to the 'Bulky Baggage' counter, and other passengers might have thought it most likely that I had checked in my washing-machine and tumble dryer.

On this particular Saturday Kira's career as a 'frequent-traveller' baby began. She was just twenty months old and a whirlwind of sunshine.

This was already her third flight. She was, of course, with us for each prior therapy. With good sense and the discipline of a 'Lady', my daughter sat for almost eleven hours, with her bottom well packed in Pampers, and occupied herself happily with every imaginable toy and plaything. Not even the endless wait of nearly four hours after landing until the customs formalities, the baggage, the wait for the bus to the rental car company and finally the collection of the car affected her. She mastered all of this quite regally. While Jaqui and I were already at our wits end, Kira was still quite content — even a Transatlantic flight was not enough to floor her — I was enormously proud of her.

Timmy too sensed that this was a very special journey. As we were both taken to the aircraft, with wheelchair, he lay in my arms, and as I took my place in this strange vehicle, I felt his tension.

But this time it was not the familiar anxious state that coursed through his limbs, or caused his breathing to become restless and his heartbeat to increase. His pulse rate increased only minimally. I think I sensed in him a combination of hope and excitement. And so I carried him, my loved one, in my arms from Düsseldorf to Key Largo.

When, at last, we finally arrived he was exhausted and pale and I had a very bad conscience for having put him through all of this.

At three o'clock in the morning the night was over for us, in spite of the time difference of six hours, the children slept a relatively long time. Key Largo lay still in darkness as we awoke in our Hotel apartment. And so we had our first early morning breakfast composed of biscuits, chocolate, tea and fruit juice. The children couldn't believe this was real. It was still dark, but their instinct told them that it should have been light long ago, and not even 24 hours ago in Düsseldorf, they needed hats and coats and here it was wonderfully warm.

I was incredibly tired, but I experienced the warm breeze, blowing in through the window, as a wonderful elixir, which awakened all my senses and gave me the feeling that there was much more life in me than I realized.

Feeling very well indeed, I stretched myself on the bed and for a moment had the desire to sleep with my husband.

Timmy dozed off again after breakfast. That calmed me, for I felt that my feeling of well-being had influenced him too. Kira played quite happily on the floor and the playthings and toys which she had brought from home gave her the confidence that everything was fine. As the sun rose we were treated to a breathtaking view of the bay.

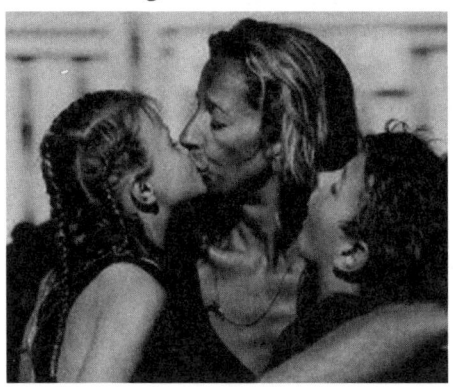

Kiki, Kira and Tim in Florida

I felt myself to be completely relaxed. In my well-practiced manner, nearly all the time with Timmy on my arm, I unpacked our goods and chattels. Our first afternoon was spent at the pool. The initiator of our journey enjoyed the warmth. Just like a sponge soaks up water, he soaked up the sunshine. But an attempt to lie him alone on the sunbed did not work, he immediately became anxious and his limbs stiffened, only becoming calm again when he was back in my arms and I gently sang to him. Kira took over the pool with her water-wings and by evening was delightfully tired.

The next morning total chaos broke out. We were all very nervous indeed and by the time we all sat in the car to drive to the therapy center we all could have each gone mad at least twice, not least of all because there was only one toilet and one bathroom in our apartment and the co-ordination, with time pressing, was difficult.

The nervous tension transformed into happy expectation, as Dr Nathanson welcomed us at Dolphins Plus. The happy, hearty and gentle manner with which he approached Timmy was a happy sight compared to some of the experiences we had had in similar situations in Germany.

'Hi ,Timmy, how are you son — I bet we'll soon be friends.' For Kira, too, he had happy words of greeting 'And who are you young lady? You must be Kira, right? Welcome to Key Largo!'

He was interested to hear that Jaqui came from Ireland and helped us and gave us support as a nurse. Dr Dave put his arms around my husband and me as if we were already the oldest of friends. 'Good to see you, how was your trip?'

A big 'Hello' started all round. We were introduced to the therapists, the secretary, the dolphin trainers and the person who took care of the little patients' little brothers and sisters. Although there were three other seriously ill patients there on this Monday morning, for the start of their therapies, the atmosphere was happy, hearty and almost relaxed. Everyone ran around like ants, but with such devotion to duty that the whole thing worked tranquilly.

Needless to say from all the different names I heard that first day, I have only managed to retain the most important ones. Dr Dave, naturally, Lou Ellen, Timmy's therapist, an attractive young lady with the blonde hair of an angel, Marcia, at that time Lou Ellen's assistant, and Elizabeth, a humorous American teenager who was responsible for the siblings of the little patients who were not only taken care of during the therapy sessions, but also had a lot of fun. This was what made it possible for the parents, free of any worries about their other children, to concentrate on the therapy sessions. Lou Ellen, Marcia, Jaqui and I prepared Tim for his first session on the dock. There were life jackets and belts to be tried and fitted — what were the best floating aids for him, which would not handicap him in the water, which were the best and most comfortable for him? Because of his spastic condition the putting-on and taking-off presented problems.

The choice of the therapists was something which looked rather like a swimsuit with air pockets, a very individual blue garment. Lou Ellen told me that she wanted to carry Timmy to the dock. With a smile and shake of the head I made it clear to her that although the happy greeting-ceremony had been great, it was not sufficient grounds to let them take my child from me. Possibly he would turn blue because, out of fear and anxiety, he would forget to breathe. When I understood — when it was quite clear to me — that Timmy could not take part in a therapy session on my arm, I felt instantly unwell. I hadn't thought of, or even considered, this fact.

Dr Dave allowed this time, as an exception, my presence on the dock, but how would we continue the next day? During the time of all other therapies I had spread my wings like a broody hen over my child so that at any time I could immediately take over control. I was neither prepared nor willing to take away my hand — the connection between us — which was always in

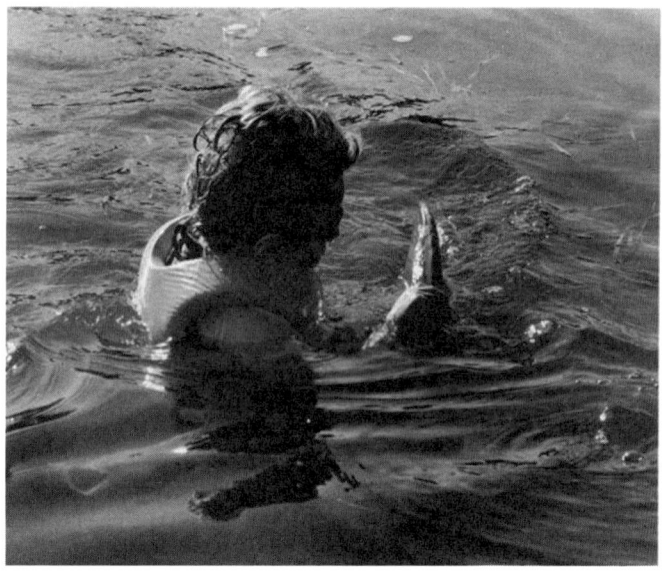

Tim has total confidence and strength

contact with some part of his body. There were only a very few people, to whom, to date, I had felt happy enough about and was able to entrust Timmy, knowing that he trusted them and therefore was not frightened or anxious. I saw now a 'battle of wills' approaching and it was not clear for whom it would be worst, for me or my son.

With a combination of love, and determination, the Dolphin Therapist took my child from my arms. Her look said to me 'Don't worry, I'll take the very best care of him'.

And so it was, for Timmy, atypically, let himself be carried away on the spell of her melodic voice, even though her language was foreign to him. The gentle stroking and the sing-song tones told him that he needed to have no fear of anything unpleasant, rather that he was in safe and capable hands.

Needless to say, he was not really completely relaxed, but the calming aura of the whole scenario seemed to touch him. He breathed regularly and was prepared to face the current situation. That reduced my fear.

I was now quite certain that he had understood all I had told him about the Dolphins and the therapy, and from my perspective, how important this was for him.

As for me, I was far from being relaxed in any way. Each and every fibre of my entire body felt as if they were electrified. With the eyes of an eagle I followed Timmy in each and every movement. I watched the fascinating playfulness of the Dolphins, these creatures whose sheer beauty is not surpassable. With her gentle disposition Dingy, a female Dolphin, tried carefully to attract Timmy's attention. If on this first day she was able to reach his soul, I cannot say. I saw no recognizable sign or reaction to the dolphin's beautiful play. I think she captured his mother more than Timmy, and almost selfishly I let myself be taken in — our eyes met in silent contact and I communicated my thanks that she was there and for her great care and efforts with my baby. She gave me something, which to this day, I could never express to anyone in words.

Lou Ellen and Marcia very cautiously made their approaches to Timmy. Playfully they tried to find out where he found himself at this time, whether he could understand them — and how they could, together, break down the wall which separated him from the rest of the world. Quickly they recognized that this barrier was almost insurmountable, but they gave the impression that this merely spurred them and motivated them to engage all possibilities to free Timmy from his isolation.

I thought of Meike Weitemeier, who was the one individual from the bank of 'professionals' who had encouraged me to undertake this trip, and who had not just laughed at me.

On our first visit to her in Hamburg, she told me that she thought Timmy was like an angel. Even when therapists should really protect themselves against such expressions of feeling or giving special attention to particular patients, she admitted that she was sure that Timmy would cast his spell upon many people and those who would allow themselves to be spellbound would certainly do their very best for him.

Quite clearly the two American therapists were at the point of falling in love with him. Their games with him had something which was almost everyday, familiar and natural, that went without words. They talked to him as old friends do, and more importantly, they treated him as a normal healthy child.

Nevertheless, in spite of all efforts, Timmy remained apathetic. He showed no interest at all either in the various playthings and took no notice of the ball, not to mention his swimming-therapist, Dingy.

The first appointment, the orientation session, was quickly over. On the other hand it had seemed to me like a lifetime, compared to all the thoughts that raced through my head, torn backwards and forwards between happiness, disappointment, magic and hope.

The first two days of the therapy followed their course without any spectacular happenings — there were no noticeable changes. However, surprising in itself, Timmy had no problem in leaving my arms and giving himself over to the care of Lou Ellen and Marcia. Without any further discussion I received permission to remain on the dock during the therapy sessions.

On the third day the time was now ripe for the first motherly intervention in the course of the session. I had fought with myself because I did not want to disturb the motivated and positive atmosphere. Nevertheless I felt that I had not brought Timmy all the way to America just to learn to listen to a rattle, to feel forms and shapes or to hum children's songs, rather for one and only reason — to make meeting and swimming with the dolphins possible. The actual contact with the dolphins did not seem to me to receive enough emphasis of its true value.

That a clear therapeutic concept lay behind the work of Dolphin Human Therapy was not quite clear to me at this point. It was not clear to me and at that time did not interest me. I wanted to see my child in the water. I wanted Dr Dolphin to do his stuff. The rest, I thought, I could have done at home.

It was really surprising that Dr Nathanson did not immediately explode when I explained my sentiments. I was in the process of questioning the concept that he had successfully discovered and built up over many years of research. You can't imagine what the result would have been if I had behaved this way with the doctors in Germany. But Dr Dave?

He listened to me, with his baseball-cap askew on his head, more than relaxed. My arguments that we could not 'reach' Timmy this way and that the 'foot-kisses' of the dolphins were not the conception of dolphin therapy that I had, that the therapists were wonderful but that I thought that one should leave the 'commanding' to the dolphins. He replied simply, 'We'll give it a try, perhaps you are right'. It was as if my dream had taken over — on the fourth day, Timmy spent almost forty minutes in the water.

Lou Ellen became Timmy's 'swimming lifejacket'. For reasons that I couldn't immediately understand, after the second session, Dr Dave had chosen Spunky as swimming therapist instead of Dingy. She was another female dolphin who brought her 13 month old son Duke to the sessions with her and showed him 'what a good therapy-dolphin must be capable of!'.

In his whole manner Duke reminded me somehow of Timmy when he was still a healthy child. He was a little rascal. 'Hey, I can do that too — let me — can I join in?' Often Spunky had to gently bring him back under control, when he got a little 'too big for his boots'. Meredith, this beautiful young dolphin trainer with a Cuban background, had her hands full making sure that the little rascal didn't bring the session into chaos with his tricks!

Marcia threw balls and rings from the docks in an attempt to attract Tim's attention, but that didn't interest him much. Blissfully he let himself cruise through the water in the arms of Lou, drawn by his new-found silvery friend Spunky and accompanied by his cheeky playmate Duke.

Obviously lightened, carried by the warm saltwater, Timmy allowed himself, without any protest, to be propelled through the water by Spunky, pushing on his foot. Sometimes I was sure that I saw the shadow of a smile fleeting across his face. Spunky never ever took her eyes off Timmy, whatever they were doing, in order that she, too, should not miss any single motion.

In the meantime the aura in the Center, the sunshine and the atmosphere of the sessions, at times allowed me to let myself go.

Kira was quite content. She had only one single problem, and that was that she, too, wanted to be close to the dolphins.

Timmy was quite well too, taking into consideration his present state. Even today sometimes I ask myself for whom this visit to Key Largo was of most benefit, for Timmy or for myself? It warmed my heart to see that he at least no longer was riddled with cramp. Even when, up till now, no spectacular change in his condition was visible, I knew that he soaked up that which the dolphins were in a position to give him.

Strength, energy, feeling, vibrations and signals — all of that which we are not perhaps able to comprehend.

And then the first of a thousand little miracles happened on Timmy's 'Journey of Hope' with the dolphins towards a better world. Suddenly at the end of the usual forty minute session, my son was in the water and Spunky pushed his foot as if to say 'Let's go boy!'. TIMMY LAUGHED LOUDLY. He laughed, he really laughed, no question. He laughed, and he laughed, laughed out loud, and squealed for joy!!!!!!

Even before his laughter stopped I WEPT — I ran from the dock, I don't know why, I ran and wept and wept. I found myself wrapped in the arms of a man I didn't know, the father of a little Welsh girl, who didn't want to calm me down — for as he held me he whispered to me that he too had witnessed everything that had just happened — 'Incredible, just incredible — how far must we travel just to experience such moments. Incredible.'

He laughed, he's back again. Timmy's back, he really laughed.

I just couldn't believe it. He laughed. He truly and really laughed.

He is happy and he is having fun, he knows that he's still alive, he's here, he laughed!

Jaqui, who had only worked with us for three weeks had glassy eyes.

Kira was agitated and didn't know why I was suddenly crying.

'Mami is so happy 'Püppi', Mami is so unbelievably happy. Timmy laughed, he's back again, your brother is back again.' With a serious face she looked at me, she had understood everything, perhaps not completely, but following the therapy she ran directly to Timmy and kissed him — and as she kissed him he smiled.

It seemed as if I was 'pass the parcel'. I was in the arms of everyone present and still I cried. Everyone held me and hugged me; strangers, parents, therapists, children, helpers and trainers. Those who had seen and heard for themselves cried with me, and the others said over and over again 'Unbelievable, a miracle' ... Lou Ellen, Marcia and I fell into each others arms and Lou wept too, Marcia discreetly wiped her eyes. They all ran back and forth between Timmy and me. 'Good boy — unbelievable, a miracle.'

Yes, that's exactly what it was, a miracle. After exactly one year, four months and eight days Spunky had awakened Timmy from his coma.

At last, I could take Timmy into my arms. He was completely exhausted and his eyes were closed. I held him as close to me as I could — I could have squeezed him to death out of sheer joy — once more I cried for happiness and whispered in his ear how happy I was, how proud I was of him, what a strong boy he was, and how immeasurably wonderful it is that he exists. For the first time in almost a year and a half his little body felt soft.

It was the day Michael came.

I felt sorry for my husband on that evening when I told him of all that had happened. That afternoon he had driven to the airport to pick up our friend, who had business in Florida and wanted to use the opportunity to pay us a visit. My husband appeared very sad that he had not been able to witness that fantastic moment himself. 'Papi, Mami crying', said Kira to add weight to the moment. It seemed to trouble her very much even though I had told her that grown-ups sometimes simply cry for happiness. I have always tried to avoid confronting my daughter with my sometimes dark and depressive emotions, and prevented myself from letting her see my often secretly-cried tears.

I called home, everyone should hear the good news. My mother was not exactly over the moon and I was disappointed. Her reaction seemed strange to me. Four days later, when we also had a not-too-happy call I put my spoke in the wheel. 'I'm at the other end of the world, do you hear me? It was the right thing to do bringing Timmy to Florida. Timmy has succeeded in taking a step back into our world. Mami, I am so happy, can't you even give me the feeling that you are happy for me — happy for Timmy?'

She seemed detached, and with almost no emotion she said she was sorry that I had the impression that she was not happy for me, but she was very tired.

Silly cow!!! — I thought to myself, and swept the conversation away.

I wasn't going to let anything or anyone in the world ruin this intense feeling that you could almost call happiness.

From here on, with every session, Timmy made tiny little steps of progress, little bats of the eyelids, but recognizable. The weekend was free of therapy and for the first time since the accident, I could lie him down by himself. He opened his hands and looked at the world with great big eyes. I felt quite lost without my 'Siamese twin' on my arm. He, at this moment, was lying on a normal sunbed and looking quite relaxed at the poolside of the Marriott Hotel in Key Largo.

After a week my husband had to fly back to Germany and left us alone. Very important business! What in God's name had to happen to make clear to him that there are situations in life where even the most important appointment crumbles into insignificance. And that in such circumstances 'being there for one another' is the be-all and end-all, the most important thing in the world. I couldn't understand.

The dear Lord God had certainly gone to a lot of trouble, and had, for all of those who had been present on that tragic day, and who shouted their grief to all and sundry, thought out a very special message. But no one had understood that Timmy had given them the opportunity to change.

Even though I was in conflict with God, due to the fact that He had tried to take my child from me, I understood, fairly early on, that what was behind this tragedy was an assignment. I was determined, if obstinately, to rise to the challenge, to accept it — for under no circumstances would I let my child be taken from me. For this was not the end, it was the beginning of a new, another life.

Saying goodbye to my husband at the airport was not easy. I didn't want him to leave and I didn't want to be without him. I truly could not understand that he did not have the strength to set his priorities and therefore, at least this time, ignore his so-called business duties. He would have only needed to say 'My family needs me now. There is nothing more important to me than to be here with my wife, my daughter, and most of all with my son.' But he went. Perhaps for that reason I found it only fair that I had been the one allowed to hear Timmy laughing.

With the same aircraft that carried my husband away from us, Barbara Schweitzer arrived in Florida. It was she who, six months previously, discovered, in the newspaper, a tiny article about Dolphin-Assisted Therapy, and had so discovered the address of Dr Dave.

Before I could even greet her properly it just all gushed out of me, 'He laughed, I'm telling you Barbara he really laughed. Oh by the way don't call me Mrs Kuhnert, I'm Kiki. What can I tell you, I hardly believe it myself. He laughed really loud.'

Our little apartment was like a camping site. Timmy 'resided' with me in the 'big bed', Kira, Jaqui and Barbara shared the second bedroom and Michael slept on the couch. For the first time in his life something was more important than his job. It was Kira who opened her little world for him and we wanted to spend a pleasant hour at the hotel pool after Timmy's therapy. Michael protested loudly that he really had to work, there were a hundred faxes to be read and phone calls to be made to Germany, Japan and the rest of the world.

Kira looked at him and simply said 'Micky, please, swimming pool'.

Well that was it — the top manager gave things no further thought, took Kira's hand and marched off with her to the pool. Barbara and Jaqui remarked on this with very knowing grins.

Kira had wound Mr Big Guy around her little finger, and, together with her brother, re-arranged his list of priorities. After two days the only adult man in our midst, each and every evening insisted that on the very next day he must return to Germany. But he also was captured by the happenings around Timmy and the dolphins, and sensed, by instinct, how thankful I was to him for his presence. And so he stole as much time as he could to spend with us, until there really was no choice.

Being room-mates, all living together, gave us all the feeling of being part of a commune, and the atmosphere was almost relaxed. Within a short period of time we became a close-knit community. No one had any inclination to leave the place in the evenings even though as far as I was concerned the other three adults had a 'free-hand'. I was more than happy to stay with the 'little ones'.

I needed no baby sitter, I wanted for nothing — but no-one went — and so, often in the evenings, we were still in bathing shorts on the balcony, cooked together and drank together the odd bottle of wine. We spoke of nothing else other than Timmy, who still did not sleep the whole night through and who kept me on the go night after night, but also day by day became more composed and settled. He had us all in his hands anyway, for he was the center of attention in all our plans, our activities and our conversations.

On one such evening as we spoke for at least the hundredth time about what united us all in America, and, as that wonderful feeling of happiness came over me once again, I threw into the group the following thought:

'Strictly speaking it should be possible for every child, who has not developed properly according to his or her age, for whatever reason, to participate in Dolphin Human Therapy.' Everyone agreed.

'But', I continued, 'who is in the position to put more than ten thousand dollars on the table "just like that" in order to pay for a two-week Dolphin-Assisted-Therapy? Somebody must form an organization, whose aim it is to make it possible that all 'special-needs' children, wherever they are, can experience this therapy.' Everyone nodded in agreement. 'You're right Kiki, and if anyone is able to bring such an organization to life, then it's you.' That was Michael's conviction and belief.

The value of hope

Surely I don't need to tell you that we left America, Key Largo, Dr Dave, Lou Ellen, Marcia, Meredith, and of course the dolphins, with very heavy hearts. It was very much more than just saying goodbye. Timmy had so positively changed, he was as brown as a bear, relaxed and happy. His hands remained opened and he suffered much less cramp. Through a very small window he seemed to be able to look into our world, and the best thing about it was that he liked what he saw.

For his mind and understanding stayed with us and his eyes watched us, even if only for a split of a second at a time. It was quite clear that he felt again how pleasant it was to have his face stroked, a ritual from old times when he was a baby, a practice I had to give up because each contact with Timmy's cheek caused intense pain. At last he could enjoy again this ritual and that was good for both our souls.

People on the outside would possibly deem me mad when I say that Timmy's health had improved dramatically. Timmy had not spoken, he couldn't walk, he could not eat alone, and he was, in all ways reliant, upon our help. But he had laughed, laughed out loud.

The features of his face had relaxed and quite simply Timmy was doing much better. I had benefited, Timmy had benefited. We had chosen the right path.

Our departure from Florida was nothing more than a firm promise — the promise to return again as quickly as possible. In Key Largo, Timmy would take more steps in his development and one day possibly be fully recovered again. The high hopes with which we had flown to Florida had not been dashed, quite the contrary.

I was addicted to Dolphin Human Therapy. More, I wanted more. More for Timmy and more for all of us. In my mind I was already planning the next visit in order to make this parting a little easier.

Shortly before landing in Düsseldorf the captain gave the actual weather report 2 degrees C and rain!!!

How awful. Germany in November. Depressing enough even for people with no problems. It depressed me and more than that, I was concerned how Timmy would deal with the change, and if the change of time zones and the change of climate would influence the great steps forward his health had taken, and hoped that these would not be destroyed.

Whilst I was still in baggage-claim I called Michael. 'Don't be sad, keep the Florida sunshine and the happy memories in your heart. And then things won't be so bad', he told me, but in a voice that was strangely troubled.

When we came out of customs I found my mother waiting. She looked absolutely dreadful and was clothed entirely in black. I took her in my arms and we hugged one another for a long time, and we cried all the time together. There was no need to tell me. My grandmother had died.

I couldn't get my feelings sorted, I was suddenly unbelievably sad, just when I had for the first time been able to see a glimmer of light at the end of the long tunnel, why now? Did I not have the right to keep my positive feelings for a little longer? Must I get another kick in the head?

It was all so unfair. I felt like a child who had been misused by life, or by destiny or whatever one chooses to call it. I wanted my grandmother back again, and Timmy should be healthy again and my husband not so distanced and the sun should shine — and who the hell had said I must grow up and be adult? I was cold.

Feeling spiteful did not help. This time too, or as I felt yet again, it was no bad dream but the naked reality that I had to face up to. I felt ashamed of myself. My grandmother had lain dying as I had spoken with my mother and the time I was abrupt with her my grandmother was no longer there. The family had agreed not to tell me anything, because they were sure that I would have packed my bags and returned home immediately. It was their wish that Timmy should continue his therapy to the very end and not to endanger this with the devastating news.

At that time I did not know whether to be grateful for this or not.

My grandmother had gone forever and I would have loved to have seen her one more time before she died. Perhaps it was the right thing after all because it was for Tim's sake. It was for his progress and his return into our world. And with this in my mind I found the family's decision the right one.

The day of her funeral was the same day as her 80th birthday. I had never imagined that I still had the capacity to cry so bitterly. The soothing words of other mourners just got on my nerves, the blithe comments 'Perhaps it was better so, — she would only have suffered. It was a great age' — and so on. When someone you deeply love takes leave, at whatever age, it's still too soon.

I was in a terrible state and was frightened that this would rub off on Timmy. The bond between us both was so strong that my state of mind always was perceived by him. But the miracle continued.

Timmy remained stable. With quite unbelievable sensitivity and great love, Barbara adjusted to the change in Timmy's condition and through this was responsible, that in a cold and frosty Germany, he lost none of his new found balance.

Barbara herself developed rapidly. Within a short period of time she became an accomplished therapist — and that not only for Timmy. In Key Largo she too had experienced something that far exceeded the bounds of normal professional experience. So, soon, it was that

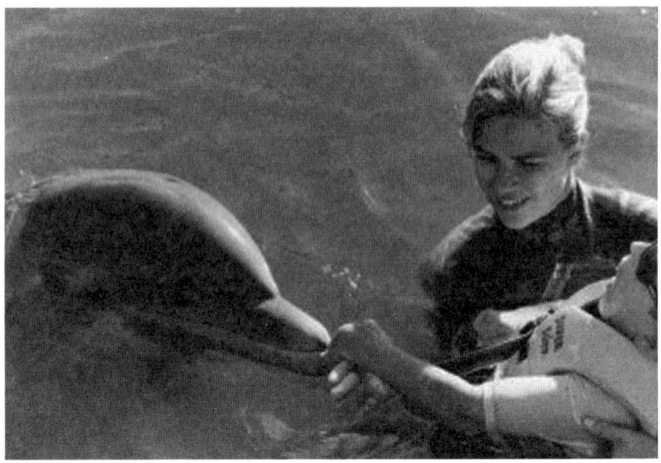

Barbara and Tim during a therapy session

Timmy did things for Barbara that he would do for no one else, and so sometimes we said 'Now, come on, do it for Babala' — that was the name Kira had given her — and also the name we still use today.

Besides all the wonderful memories, I had brought something else important with me back from Key Largo. What had Michael said? 'When someone has the ability to call an organization to life, then that person is you'. With the reminder of these words was born the idea of forming *dolphin aid*.

In the weeks following however I had to first learn about forming such a charity. What was necessary in Germany to form a charity is a foundation for the good of the community, officially speaking. I learnt that seven members of a founding group are required, a statement of the aims and intents of the group and registration at the local courthouse. When all that is done its a case of 'off we go'. A charity which asks for donations also needs authority from the Inland Revenue department, to receive tax deductions — and this too had to be sorted out.

But first of all what about the seven forming members? Naturally Michael, if he put the idea into the world then he is part of it, like it or lump it — then myself — that left five more. Christian, my assistant from the agency, he was in it too.

And then I called my friend Biggi, that's Birgit Lechtermann with her proper name, a TV presenter for children's programs. She was immediately taken with the idea, particularly as she too had witnessed the changes in Timmy, since our return from America. To keep the whole thing 'in the family' her husband Willy Knupp also became a founding member. Number five. And then I had a quick word with Thomas and Akki, that's Dr and Dr Schierl, a media scientist and a dental surgeon. They too 'jumped into our boat'. Our logo, 'our banner', was conceived on the computer and the official meeting of the founding members organized.

As a basis for the new charity I translated all the information and material from Dr Nathanson from English into German. The charter of the new organization was to promote dolphin therapy and to advise the families of afflicted children and, when necessary, to give a helping hand and financial support.

Together we composed the charter line by line until all was in black and white on paper. Now *dolphin aid* had information material and that had to be printed. The owner of a printing works, with whom I had worked in my agency days and had received much business from me, was roped in to do this. He knew the background and was happy to help us. To this day he has never even asked for a tax relief certificate for the work he did for us, his charges waived.

The last stepping-stone was the taxman, and when the official recognition of *dolphin aid* as a not-for-profit charity was approved we were 'Ready for take off'.

In the meantime the condition of 'Mr dolphin aid' himself had continually improved. Every day a little miracle.

He began to make speech noises, he ate better and he was quite happy with himself. The grisly moodiness of former times, which generally appeared around five in the afternoon and indicated 'Just let this day be over' had suddenly disappeared. The spastic condition was still apparent, but in the meantime Timmy was able to sit better, he was able to concentrate for a much longer time on something and also to follow what was going on. He surprised us each day with little steps forward. The dolphins, especially Spunky and Duke and his human American therapist had smoothed his path, and shown the direction back to a better life.

Forgotten were the hours in which he writhed in pain, in which his little body was taken over by unseen forces and he was lost in a world of groaning. When after four spoonfuls of nourishing food eaten were then vomited, and the constant fear of having to feed him through a tube, which always accompanied us. Today these times seem quite unreal to me and it's sometimes as if they never happened.

And when I try as hard as I can to remember these times I realize that this form of forgetfulness is, in fact, a merciful relief. With certainty I could never survive all of that again. I could not again bear to think that on each and every day Timmy could have left us.

Spunky, a very special dolphin

Martin had freed Timmy from the valley of death and brought him back to life. But it was really Spunky who brought Timmy back to 'our world' and released him from part of his isolation. For that reason I feel the same degree of thanks and love for her that I do for the original life-saver. She will always remain for me something very, very special.

But how can one describe a relationship with a friend with whom you cannot share a glass of wine, a cup of coffee or with whom you can't smoke a cigarette?

That which binds Spunky and me is the highest form of communication, namely that without words.

Our relationship is never on an even level because she understands me better than I understand her. I can't fool her. She has the ability to see through me. Even with the best make-up she recognizes my inner self. Her all-seeing eyes are able to see into the very depths of my soul and she sees it all. Little indications, explanations and enormous feelings, which in the course of the years I have learnt from her, just being in her presence. Just from sitting there and being near her.

I have often told her 'That's right, my dear, you are the better mother for Timmy'. She knows right away when and where he has a problem. I need a little longer than she does. She just simply knows when something is wrong with Timmy, and no one needs to tell her.

When I think of her I remember so many beautiful experiences.

First and foremost that Thursday in Key Largo when she made Timmy laugh and thereby 'woke him up'. The start of a new life.

Over and over again she impressed me anew, with each meeting.

I can remember many incidents through which I became certain that she was not only able but willing to take over the therapy command here and there. For example following an operation on Timmy's right hip he was extremely sensitive on his legs, most particularly the right. Things which he had enjoyed doing in the past were then not possible simply because it was painful.

One key factor which marks the dolphin therapy in Key Largo is that the animals have been taught what they should not do during a therapy session. In order not to frighten the children these clever water-therapists have learnt never to approach from behind.

As soon as Spunky realized that Timmy's foot was painful when she touched him she just turned the tables and from then on gently prodded his back or played on his neck and they glided gently through the water. Her eyes were always fixed on the Boss, her trainer Meredith, to decide whether or not there would be trouble when she took things into her own hands. Meredith, who was usually always quick-witted and ready with the right cool order for her dolphins, was moved in the same way as others who looked on. She allowed Spunky a free hand in the safe knowledge that this very special dolphin lady knew exactly what she was doing. Often she was the mother who could do more for Timmy than I could.

Then, in the course of the therapy sessions, the problems that he had following the operation were eased, thanks to Dr Spunky.

The first time I had the chance to go into the water with Spunky, long after Timmy's first therapy, I experienced such an indescribable feeling that I could have completely forgotten the rest of the world. I felt practically weightless, as if this dolphin, for a fraction of a second, had relieved me of all my worries, and shown me the lighter side of life. She drew me through the water and transported me into a state comparable to nothing else in the world and one which is addictive. I played with her in the way I had played as a child and she taught me to laugh again with all my heart.

How does one thank a lady friend who can't put flowers in a vase or who finds the smell of Chanel No. 5 unpleasant? Only with the heart. Spunky is the friend who never asks what she will receive.

She just simply gives.

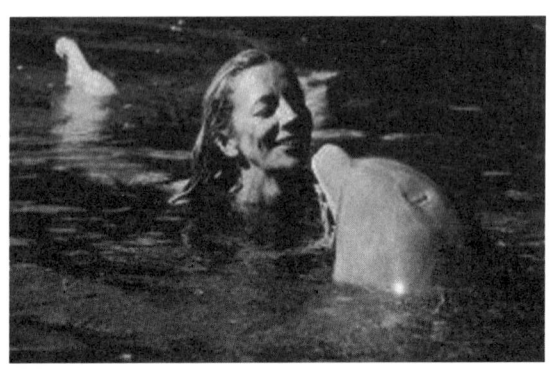

The ease of being

She gave her friendship also to Kira. At the age of only three my daughter swam alone with Spunky and Duke with an absolute confidence in these huge playmates. Often Spunky simply took her out into her own world and almost didn't want to bring her back to us. The dolphins have adopted Kira as a dolphin-child, and that she is with body and soul.

I remember a very special episode involving Michael and Spunky, which by the way would make a good story for a film or cartoon. Michael arrived in Key Largo suffering from jet lag, overworked and irritable. I remember exactly it was Thanksgiving and we were practically alone at Dolphins Plus. I asked my good friend, the head trainer Rudolf, to simply throw Michael into the water with Spunky, before I did something more drastic myself. Michael lamented that he didn't want to and apart from that he didn't have any shower stuff with him, and so on. After about half an hour Spunky had achieved that which courses for 'overstressed businessman' usually need four weeks to do. Michael was a changed person. His eyes were bright and sparkling and he was relaxed and in the best of moods.

To whomsoever asks me how swimming with the dolphins affects you, I always quote this incident. When it's possible that a man ruled by just common sense can be transformed within the space of thirty minutes into another person, and that this transformation is the result of an experience which is not able to be explained through pure logic, then it's quite clear what potentials lie within this therapy.

When people close to me come to visit in Florida to see for themselves the reason I turn down invitations, refuse parties and sacrifice my private life, I always introduce them first of all to Spunky and her son Duke. After this experience no one ever asks the same questions again as before.

I have observed in healthy strangers human reactions which have captured me and a few which have made me knowingly grin. Women who left the water with tears streaming down their cheeks due to the sudden appearance of a flood of feelings. Or the 'macho' men, whom I have seen after a date with Spunky, who were transformed into 'gentle-men'.

Because of our fantastic experiences that we have had with the dolphins and especially the therapy, Tim, Kira and I try, in spite of the enormous costs involved — each therapy trip costs about US$12,000 — to travel at regular intervals to Florida.

When my ex-husband announced a visit to us, after about three years, I had a very funny feeling. For the sake of my children I did not want his visit to cause friction and wanted just to have a peaceful pleasant time.

As I was not able to judge his mood or his intentions in advance I planned for the first day of his visit a trip to Dolphins Cove, a new therapy center, where Spunky had found a new home. I was sure that she would be the best ally I could wish for. It did not need a secret phone call to tell her how she could positively influence my ex-husband, nor to tell her of my anxieties. As ever I could rely upon her. He came out of the water, and for a moment I thought I saw the man again with whom I had fallen in love a long time ago.

He was happy and relaxed and had on his face that old cheeky grin, that I had always so loved, just like a young lad who had just had an extraordinary experience. After this we spent a few really enjoyable and, most of all, harmonious days together.

Whenever I'm having a bad time I always think of Spunky, and on that which she did for my child. I think how lucky I am that she exists. And whenever it's possible I swim with her, even if it is sometimes only for a few minutes. Then it is as if someone had recharged my empty batteries.

Quite normal madness

Following Timmy's accident I tried, for quite a while, in a show of strength, to continue operating my sport promotion agency. Our life was geared to be, up until then, wherever possible, successful in the business world. We had taken on financial responsibilities which we could afford, because both my husband and I were doing well in business. However my instinct already told me at the end of that fatal year 1994 that I could not survive this multiple stress for any length of time.

With the founding of my agency I had transformed my passion for motor sport into a career. In this way I wanted to lay down my future professionally and to have an alternative to my much loved 'Job in the Clouds', of which I would not want to have missed a single moment. But the examples of cabin staff, at some stage left high and dry, attempting to find the way back to a normal routine life with an eight to five job, are without number. I wanted to shield myself from this happening to me and therefore formed the agency 'Sponsoring Consulting' — with the aim to being able to, in the future, make my own schedule, and that for the benefit of my children.

With an enormous portion of luck in this business, which is usually a man's world, I soon found myself playing in the upper league. And for that reason my clients and partners were quite used to me putting 200% of myself into my projects. In spite of home, husband and children this was, for me, more pleasure than problem.

We traveled to the races, which were mostly held at the weekends. as a group with a big mobile home, to be on base in the paddock, the 'Timmymobile' so that even though I had many appointments and meeting after meeting, I was still able to play my mother role, and always have Timmy near me.

It was clear from the beginning that I would not be a woman who, upon finding herself pregnant, started to only then think in terms of nappies and babies' bottles.

I was a mother with body and soul but I owed it to myself, my husband and I owed it to my children not to become a frustrated housewife.

After Timmy's accident, when I thought out loud about my future and the obvious need to close the agency so that I could devote myself entirely to Timmy and Kira, my husband's casual response only was to enquire 'And how do you imagine we are going to keep things going then?'.

It was more than a year later, after the collapse of our marriage, that I was in a position to make my own decision on this point. In the meantime I had continued — without those around me noticing — on the edge of a nervous breakdown, daily.

My everyday tasks were so organized that any fairly normal person would have needed a week to cope with them all. I was not just turning at full revolutions I was permanently overtaxing the engine. Nevertheless each evening I still had the feeling that I had not done enough.

My marriage broke down in the most hideous way. And to answer the question if Timmy's accident was responsible for that, I can directly reply: 'NO! That was not it. And I cannot even claim that my husband left me.

The reason is in fact quite simple. Our relationship was already on the rocks before Kira's birth. We had both missed the chance to develop together, to learn to adjust to each other and to understand one another. We just simply drifted apart. And a tragedy like that which happened to our son unquestionably brings two people to the brink of their tolerance. There is no chance to sweep things under the carpet, then the differences are too obvious. When the point arrived where we no longer just attacked one another verbally to find an outlet for our despair over Timmy and to compensate ourselves, I had to reach a decision. Should I consume the rest of my energy on the battlefield of my marriage, use it on a husband who I still loved but who, quite obviously, could not give me the love and support, the warmth and attention that I needed?

I made a decision and that was to be there for my children; so that Kira could become a happy young girl, and to give Timmy every possible assistance and encouragement.

What I didn't know by that time was that I had chosen a pretty stony path. But this soon became crystal clear to me. Even though the path I chose carried me to places I had not known existed before, I am still today certain I made the right decision. Neither the path to the welfare offices or to the pawn-shop, none of the discrimination or the bad gossip and also not the friends who have been lost along that way could have ever held me back from my goal.

The energy which I gained from the love of my children was far stronger than any experience which robbed me of my dignity. I have gone through this terrible time, with daily attacks on my nervous system and on my emotions not only with my head held up high, but with complete honesty to myself. And the recognition that, when I think about Timmy, how everything else sinks into a state of worthlessness, has given me a degree of personal freedom that I had never imagined I would achieve.

What could drive me off the rails today? A sick child? I have one. A separation? I've done that one. Having to sell my jewelry? There is not much left anyway. Applying for welfare? I was already there. Go to a pawn shop? I know it, it's not located at the best address. Have to go to the doctor? Should do so. Have no money? That's quite normal and everyday. Disappointment in other humans? Thanks, I've had enough already.

Had I had sensed into which tracks my life would fall in trying to realize what I thought was my life's dream — husband, marriage, children, a happy world, home and family, leaning on the garden fence — it's for sure I would have run a mile.

Perhaps though, I would have been spared the deepest wounds — this pain which knows no boundaries and is always there deep inside me which sometimes robs me of the will to live and takes my breath away.

But I believe there are no coincidences. So in December 1995 *dolphin aid* existed, founded in a naive way, based on the wish to help, in a small way, one brick at a time. And suddenly it was an avalanche. The first article appeared in the newspaper.

As a result the TV channel SAT 1 called me. Germany's most famous talk show host wanted me to appear as a guest in her show.

What followed I can hardly describe. Naively I had given my private phone number. The phone just didn't stop ringing any more. *dolphin aid* had started and it was a pretty steep take-off.

Although my sponsoring agency no longer actively existed, I still worked in every free minute, up to sixteen hours a day, constantly into the early hours of the morning and especially in the time my mother thought I would have done better to relax. I followed an inner urge, possibly connected with the intense desire to transform the blow that fate had dealt my son in some way, into something meaningful and of value.

And once again a little miracle happened. In the course of hundreds of phone calls with other parents I learnt that I was not the hardest done-by on this Earth. There were stories which moved me to tears, and situations that I would never have conquered. Death penalty situations for children — and their parents were damned to be spectators in this senseless scenario.

I sat and manned the phone for *dolphin aid* and sensed how the people at the other end of the line relaxed and let themselves go during the course of our conversations. And suddenly I was the one giving courage. Timmy had thought out for me a very special way of coping with my own trauma. Through his development and especially through the visits to the dolphins he had enabled me to do that which I had missed most myself — to be a good listener, to comfort, counsel, help and quite simply to be there for others.

The calls echoed into one another, giving me the energy for the next one, and the one after that. No phone call was shorter than an hour.

Within only a few weeks I was no longer able to cope with the flood of enquiries. I would only be away for a couple of hours with Timmy for therapy and upon my return the voice mail on my cell phone and the answering machine were full of messages. Many parents seeking help will well remember that sometimes my first call-back to them was at a time when most people are in bed and I had to permanently excuse myself that I risked calling strangers shortly before midnight. All had full understanding for my odd office hours when I explained to them that Timmy had only just fallen asleep and that it was possible I would have to interrupt the conversation to attend to him. With some people I clamped the phone to my ear while seeing to Timmy, when his cries called me to his room.

I desperately needed help, and my activities for *dolphin aid* could not be allowed to burden the children, so I worked principally at night which did not do a lot for my state of health. My constant lack of sleep left me with rings like a racoon. Daily I waited in the fear that someone might say 'Gosh Mrs Kuhnert for a fifty year old you've kept well!!!!'.

The greatest difference to my former work was quite clear — I no longer wrote invoices for the work I had performed. Much later on a very nice man at the bank said to me 'Mrs Kuhnert, all the charity work you do, all well and good, but don't you think it's about time you did some work for money'. He possibly could not understand how someone who had a bank statement like mine could sleep at nights.

But in the end he was always most understanding, and without his help I would most likely have been shipwrecked and bankrupt in my attempts, ten times over. It was he who made sure that I was not taken for a potential bank robber when I used my ATM bank card.

The first travel group organized by *dolphin aid* set off in October 1996 to Miami. Tour leader, donation-beggar, psychiatrist, organizer, counsellor and interpreter were all combined in one person — me. On top of all this I had to fulfil my responsibilities as a mother of a severely handicapped son and a two year old baby girl.

Already in this first group there was a child whose entire costs, travel and therapy, had been paid for by

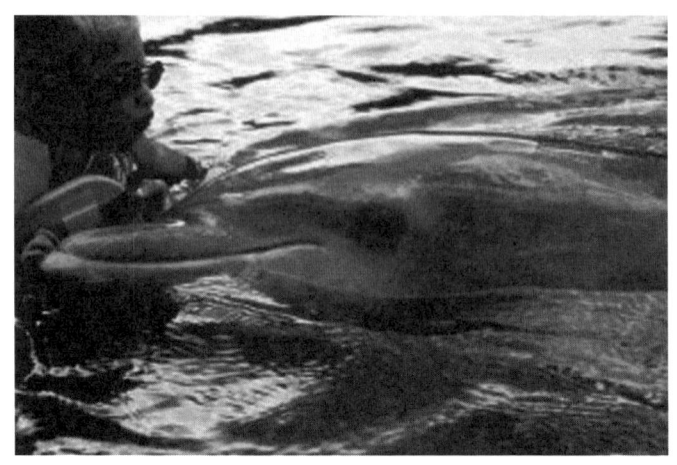

The joy of working with the dolphins

dolphin aid. For that reason I called my friend Ulli in Essen and told him that there was a family with a 'special needs' child. The mother was bringing up her child alone and that there were also three other kids, that they all lived together in a tiny flat, and so on. And so it was that Ulli, who has a heart of gold, became the first big benefactor for *dolphin aid*.

Naturally I had previously spoken with my old friend and colleague Karl Hermann Hansen from the LTU Press and Public Relations Department and asked about, for one family or another, the possibility of free flights to Miami.

He promised that it was a matter of honor, or so, for him, he spoke with his boss and from 'A few tickets for a family' resulted lots of tickets for eight families, and the staff at LTU promised to do anything they could to help in the course of their duties to make things smoother for these travelers.

The Public Relations Department organized a separate check-in counter for us and it was arranged that all the members of our undertaking would be brought to the aircraft in a separate bus. With a TV crew and photographers we departed, well taken care of, for Miami.

We picked up the reserved rental cars at the Alamo station at Miami airport and drove in a convoy in the direction of Key Largo. Adventure from the first moment on, that could well have been our slogan.

All these pioneer families of the first trip have repeated their therapies with their children during the past few years. For without exception each and every child had made great progress during the first therapy trip, thanks to Dr Dolphin and thanks to Dolphin Human Therapy, one little boy, Darius, even began to walk.

Lukas's mother, Maria Börner, who is today one of my very best friends, came to me at the pool, her tears streaming, 'He looked at me, he looked at me deep into my eyes, for the first time ever'.

Bernhard who through spastic problems had never in his life been able to use his right arm came out of the water after his therapy, went to the shower — and turned on the water — with his right hand!!!

There were so many moving moments that we often had to reach for our tissues. Often in the evenings I took Timmy in my arms and told him, 'Hey, that's you, you've done all that, you made it possible. You have made sure that so many people could laugh, and some cry again today, simply because they are happy.' Then he would look gently into my eyes and there was a little grin on his face. **Every day a little miracle.**

A charity grows

In the search for a pastor who would conduct our marriage ceremony — for I wasn't even baptized — we came into contact with Matthias Heimer.

His complete openness, his rhetoric and theatrical gestures captured everyone who listened to him, such that he preached to full or overfilled churches. Even my agnostic family, whose stomachs almost turned at the thought of a visit to church, were taken with this man, who in the pulpit preached with such vigor and energy that one sat in fear that the whole church would collapse onto the ground!

From the very beginning we conversed deeply, discovering ourselves to be 'brothers in soul'. And I can imagine no subject whatsoever about which he had no opinion or nothing to say. A cosmopolitan, he grew up in Athens, speaks perfect Greek and other languages, with the spiritual career of a Samaritan in the sense of the word, a wonderful listener and a sensitive counsellor.

Following the wedding we naturally remained in touch and it doesn't need to be said where our children were baptized, first Timmy, and then two years later, Kira.

Matthias came to us on the same day as the accident at the Intensive Care Unit. No one knows to this day who had told him. Even when he could not in the remotest way help me, it was the gesture that counted. We became friends.

I have often spoken with him in the moments of my deepest despair.

About the 'why?'. To this there is no answer, that we both knew.

We have philosophized about God, the paths our lives take, whether the blows of fate we receive lead us to interpret them as a task which we find the strength to master, or whether this is the solution we find to make things easier.

For these very reasons it was close to my heart to seek his help and support for *dolphin aid*. And once more I was lucky.

The active members working for *dolphin aid* were now Michael, Matthias and myself, but it was soon clear to us that this was not enough. We needed, at least, a doctor, a tax specialist, a psychologist, a travel co-ordinator, someone to organize the volunteers, someone to take care of all the correspondence, a sociologist, someone to deal with the media, and a press-officer. We needed sponsors, donors, patrons and, for the most part, a whole horde of helping hands.

The media fell in love with us from the beginning. Possibly it was the mixture of a mother who had been dealt this card of fate and she herself heading this little organization that appealed, for we got more attention in the media than many large and well established charities.

With thanks we accepted every possible help from the members of the media. They were our voice and at the start our only possibility to make the world aware that *dolphin aid* existed at all. Even today there is hardly ever a media exposure without a call for donations. And after numerous talk show appearances the lady cashier at my local supermarket greeted me with the words 'I saw you on TV yesterday'.

Our media documentation quickly grew from just a little folder to big thick files. The greatest compliment for *dolphin aid* was that, in most of the well researched reports, it was quite clear that the authors themselves were captivated by the material and so it was that we made it to the medical page of the *World on Sunday*, a most serious and acknowledged German Sunday paper.

Following a radio interview a listener called me to say that I had caught the imagination and feelings of a whole group of cool advertising specialists who had heard my broadcast and they wanted to know what they could do for *dolphin aid*.

From this phone call a whole new era for our charity, and a respectful friendship with the caller and his wife, began.

Dolphin aid got a new 'logo', a very professional presence, we had briefings, had meetings, discussed, sorted out, sometimes rejected and finally blessed our new 'baby'.

A great number of people were occupied designing layouts, doing lithographs, printing and so on and so forth. Everything which we, to date, have dispatched on information — material from the initial layout up to the final product, right from the text ideas, even our business cards and up to the final choice of pictures — these have all been donations. Each single card, each photo, each envelope is the result of a generous donation from some kind-hearted person to help us get on our feet.

In these start-up times many people advised us that we needed a better structure, a quality control, and a finer network. Thanks for the tip folks!!! That was quite clear to us anyhow, but how could three lonely fighters, working voluntarily, who were hardly able to keep up with sending out the requested information material also work on improved structures? And even the employment of a secretary, at that time, would have meant that three children less per year would have the chance to experience the healing meeting with the dolphins.

We were prisoners of our own ideas and I couldn't bear again to hear myself saying 'At the moment I'm pretty much in stress' because this 'moment' had already been going on for a couple of years, and to this date has not changed. And it obviously never will. It's clear to us all that we must continue nevertheless, motivated by the children who return from Dolphin Human Therapy and the descriptions and stories of their happy parents.

As the mountain of work to be done reached unbelievable proportions we had to do something. And so the charity *dolphin aid* was re-organized to its present form.

In the course of time we were able to fill all the positions we had dreamed of. Timmy had gathered together a board of directors, a five star team of highly engaged and motivated special people of whom some commercial companies would be very jealous.

In the meantime we had sixteen full members of the charity, and daily many more supportive ones. What has not changed in the course of time is the relationship between the 'main' and the part-time workers and helpers.

Even now the scenario Timmy has created is dominated by a few workaholics who are still waiting, innocent and hoping daily for better, or shall we say, quieter times. The volume of our work is considerable. In the meantime there is an assistant to the board in Germany, Mrs Roswitha Rauh, responsible for the office in Duesseldorf, who is the only single person who receives money for the work she does. Daily anew she reveals herself as a tower of strength and makes it possible for me to master all the administrative work before the year's end.

Claudia is the whirlwind who runs the office for our internal travel organization and is the internal, and voluntary, travel co-ordinator. She is a lady of the first *dolphin aid* hour and had helped me, long before joining the charity, to transport 'our families'. The children and families simply love her and she has developed into the chaotic soul of *dolphin aid*. There is hardly a journalist or photographer for whom she has not booked the accommodation. She belongs naturally to the inner circle of those I could not be without.

In the Duesseldorf office a whole bunch, a horde of volunteers, in a day's work, at various times fight their way through the jungle of applications received from all sorts of special teaching methods and students of these schools, from speech therapists, teachers of backward and handicapped children, physical and occupational therapists and doctors completing their studies as to their intentions concerning dolphin therapy. One may wish to work as a volunteer in a therapy center, the next wants to write his diploma or dissertation on the subject, others still wish to be honorary helpers for the families during their stay in Florida and so on. The flood of donation certificates, which are needed for the tax-man, together with the many enquiries which we receive asking about financial support are dealt with by Jutta. She also has to cope with all the various bills and accounts, together with maintaining the important links to the therapy centers in this respect. Tony Martin is our angel when it comes to translations. Voluntarily he transforms piles of German information into English documents.

Thorsten von der Heyde is the master of the figures. He too could not have imagined for a short time that a small boy would considerably reduce his free time. Thorsten has taken over as the treasurer of the board for *dolphin aid*. He watches over the books like an eagle. He co-ordinates with the Inland Revenue, with the authorities and the bank, takes care of the donations and the bank transfers for Germany and abroad. On the side he also does the payroll, he files away and does the archives and in the presentation of his figures is quite uncompromising. Thorsten has, himself, a handicapped sister who lives in a home. He knows exactly what it means to have a 'special' child in the family and also how it is for the brothers or sisters.

Michael steers the boat in all matters concerning marketing. All responsibilities in the area of sponsor co-ordination and event planning together with our agency BMZ in Duesseldorf, or Saleaway in Munich, who work for us without charge, the development of advertising and campaigns, the writing of material in English and the acquiring of new partners all fall within his resource. And needless to say he too does all of this voluntarily.

Dirk is a charming pediatrician from Cologne. He was introduced to me by Biggi Lechtermann, because he wanted to see for himself in Florida what Dolphin Human Therapy was all about. I remember well, it was another one of 'those' days. Timmy had therapy from morning until the evening and anyway he never slept the whole night through. Kira was still quite small and, in her urge to discover the world, could be pretty wearing. The office from *dolphin aid* was still at home and so I had to manage anyway, with little sleep. A meeting with this doctor, at present, did not really fit in with my plans. But when my friend gets an idea into her head she doesn't let go. So we met 'for an hour' with Mr Müller-Liebenau. After exactly one hour we transferred our round of talks to my home because I had no peace until I was back with my children.

Dirk and I became immediately 'one-heart and one-soul', and it was as if we had known one another for a long time. And so the evening which had begun in a bad mood ended at two in the morning, after ten times upstairs and downstairs to Timmy, but I was in the best of moods, having got to know a really nice person.

Following his return from his Florida holiday, Dirk had also been infected with the *dolphin aid* virus. Since this time, the charming pediatrician from Cologne is a member of our medical advisory team. And he is my friend.

The chairman of the medical advisory board from *dolphin aid* is Dr Jürgen Lindemann. We had our first personal meeting long before Timmy's accident. If I remember correctly, I was pregnant with Kira, and it was at a dinner party of friends. The evening ended for the others on a miserable note because Jürgen and I had discovered that we had lots of the same friends and both of us had a passion for the motorsport scene. We enjoyed ourselves enormously, but I had the impression that the others felt left out and couldn't laugh with us. It didn't seem to matter.

So I got to know, on that evening, the Porsche racing doctor about whom I had heard many interesting and funny tales. When I later spoke to him, for the first time, about *dolphin aid*, he told me that he, together with other doctors, had formed the Agitas Circle, which was a medical organization devoted to helping children from war torn zones, to operate on them without charge, to ship out hospital equipment and in this way to support hospitals in developing countries.

It seems to me that the day has more than 24 hours for Jürgen. Early in the morning he goes riding on one of his horses, then he does surgery or has consultations in his permanently overfilled practice. Apart from this he is a specialist for allergies, a sport doctor, a racing team doctor and is on the board of the aforementioned Agitas Circle. In addition he has a wonderful wife, Nicole, three great children and at the moment is engaged in writing the *Basic rules in the investigation of the results of Dolphin Human Therapy along German and European guidelines* — on the side, so to speak! He too is my friend. In moments when I don't feel good, his name comes to me.

That Barbara Schweitzer today has taken over the running of the Miami station is a logical consequence of our connection and friendship of many years. She had come a big step along the path together with Timmy and myself and also, in the past few years, her life had taken on a different form. Her close binding contact with my son resulted in the following letter, which demonstrates the depth of their bond.

'My Dearest Tim,

I am writing this letter to you in Miami. That which brought me here is a long story, and it is that story which I want to tell you. It's more than seven years ago that I first came into your room at the University clinic to meet you. You lay there in your mother's lap during the time I introduced myself as a physical therapist. You weren't at all well at the time.

I will never forget the first time we had a therapy session together.

You cried an awful lot and I felt on the brink of my emotional and professional abilities. At the beginning I had the feeling that I was not able to reach you at all, you were too far away. I didn't know at all, at that time, whether or not you could hear or understand me. Most of the time you were as stiff as a board and had over stretched yourself.

It was very important to get you out of this state. Your mother was with us during the course of the therapy, and from time to time I would send her out for a breath of fresh air, or to have a cigarette.

After a few days I finally managed to find a way through to you. I had brought with me a large medicine ball into the room and I laid you over it. I knelt down and said to you 'Tim, when you understand me, then you must raise your head'. You gathered together all of your strength and your energy and after a while you lifted your head by yourself, just a little bit. I will never ever forget that moment because it became clear to me that you had understood me.

I told the professor and everyone on the ward and they were not immediately prepared to believe me. Later during a visit we were both able to show your abilities to them.

I prayed for it to be a success. And just look at that, after our first try the professor himself knelt on the floor and asked you if, just for him, you could lift your head again. He asked — and you did it! — and all were amazed, because they had not expected such a reaction from you — but it didn't seem to change things a lot.

You were in our clinic for three weeks and in this time we built up a strong bond between us. Afterwards you came to me for therapy regularly.

One day your mother asked me if I had ever heard anything about a therapy with dolphins. I answered that I hadn't but that I would keep my eyes and ears open and see if I could gain any information. As if by chance, or was it perhaps destiny? I was leafing through a magazine in my dentist's waiting room and I suddenly found an article about dolphins in Florida. In a small corner of the article was mentioned that a Dr Nathanson worked with handicapped children and dolphins. I gave this little snippet from the magazine directly to your mother and she flew off to Florida to look at things for herself.

When she returned she was very impressed with what she had seen and had already made an appointment for you. She asked me if I would accompany you both for a week. Of course I said yes. And so my connection with Florida began.

In October 1995 you then flew to Florida, to the dolphin therapy. When I arrived a week later your mother, who was so excited, told me that you had laughed for the first time! It really was a fact that, after this stay in Florida, you were much more relaxed and could for the first time 'make yourself heard' again. This was a great step not just for you, but also for us, something very special.

It was, and is still, a moving experience to see you swimming, working and playing with your dolphins, while your mother was so impressed and inspired from this therapy she formed the charitable foundation *dolphin aid* in order to give other children the opportunity, with the help of this therapy, to take great steps forward.

Back in Germany, we both tried to give depth to that which you had learnt, and I think in the past years we have achieved a lot together. In time I gave you daily therapy. When we were not in the water we practised on the mat. For example I turned you over on to your tummy, which you didn't want to, and almost weren't able to, do at the start, and practised with you on the medicine ball. I encouraged you to stretch and also to widen and to train your sense of perception. You put a lot of effort into this and the control of your head and your sense of perception really improved. As a reward, at the end of each therapy session I wrapped you in a warm blanket, rocked you with your mother's help and sang to you the song 'Can you hear the rainworms coughing?'.

A landmark in our work together was when I was rocking you, you laughed out loud for the first time during therapy in Germany. It was such fun for you that we did not want to stop. The beautiful thing about our relationship is that we have both learnt from one another.

And so one block was built on top of the other. As you became stronger and more aware I stood you up on your feet. Supporting yourself on mattresses you made your first attempts at standing. I think it was a funny thing for you to look at the world again from above.

In the meantime there was naturally one or the other setback, caused by your hip operation or pneumonia. But after a time of practising diligently you were soon again the 'old' Tim. In the years following you flew to Florida twice a year for Dolphin Human Therapy. Other children

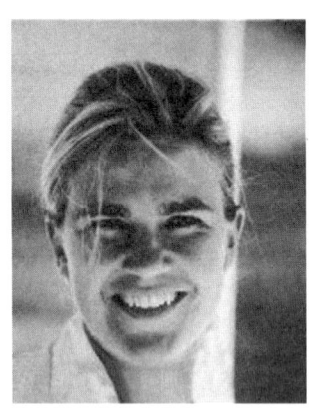

Barbara Schweitzer — Tim's therapist

at that time also gained the opportunity to meet the dolphins, with the support of your mother's charity *dolphin aid*.

In Germany we both tried to work out new steps of development, be it sitting-up, standing or practising flowing movement. Sometimes you were cross with me, seeming to say to me 'Now, that's enough!', but I had learnt, with a little firm discipline, to animate you into fighting on — even at times when it troubled my heart to do so.

I accompanied you for a long time on your regular therapy trips to the USA, until your mother asked me whether or not I wanted to become the representative of *dolphin aid* and to take care of the children and their families. Well, Tim, my dear, there I stood confronted with a big decision. I gathered together all of my courage and on February 24, 1999, flew to Miami with two suitcases.

Years have now passed. Dear Tim, looking back I have experienced so many wonderful moments through you, got to know some lovely people and gained much personal experience. Through you I found the courage to take this step, years ago that decision for me would have been quite unthinkable — I would not have had the strength. If it were not for you I would not be sitting here. Besides which I think I can, in the name of all the *dolphin aid* children, direct a very big thank-you to you, because you are there and have given them all the opportunity to experience those wonderful moments with the dolphins.

As your physiotherapist, but much more as your friend, I wish for you that you retain your bravery and your fighting spirit, that you don't give up, but that you carry on fighting, also in the moments when the courage deserts you. It's all worth it! After all it was you that showed me.

I thank you from the bottom of my heart that through you I have found the way here, and hug you close to me,
Your Babala'.

Birgit, 'Biggi' Lechtermann has been my friend for almost twenty years and, after leaving the advisory board of *dolphin aid*, Germany, has taken up the post of 'Special Ambassador' for *dolphin aid*. Whenever there are special events, conventions or other important happenings are held for the benefit of our charity, 'Biggi' is on the ball. As one who was there from the start she is a most competent interview partner.

The first Ambassador of Goodwill for *dolphin aid* and *dolphin aid America* is the internationally known racing driver, Hans-Joachim Stuck. Through my friendship with 'Stucki', which really is one of over twenty years' standing, I could tell you many tales which would fill up complete evenings! It began with my teenage idolization for this super racing driver, continued in business contact through my agency, right up to his marriage with Sylvia.

After 'Stucki' and his two sons Johannes and Ferdinand had been together in the water with Spunky, it was no longer necessary for me to ask the question as to whether or not he would take on the position of an ambassador for us. Hans-Joachim Stuck is one of the most loved German sportsmen, he is with body and soul the father of two great sons and with all his heart an ambassador for *dolphin aid*. It really is good to know that it is possible to retain a friendship over such a long time and in fact, at the end, to intensify it even further.

The crowning glory, in the true sense of the word, of *dolphin aid* is our patron, His Royal Highness Prince Leopold von Bayern.

At some stage I thought hard about who would be the ideal person to represent and to be the patron of *dolphin aid*. My demands, it proved, were pretty high. Anyway he, or she, had to be free of any scandals, believable, have both feet on the ground, and certainly the mother or father of more than one child, not be neurotic about their position, an eloquent person, be charming and also prominent.

And even if I perhaps make a *faux pas* with many wonderful people, the one single person who fulfils all of these requirements is my friend Poldi, His Royal Highness, Prince Leopold von Bayern. It's a fact that he is related to the majority of the European royal houses and a master of balance between court behavior and the smell of petrol which accompanies the international racing paddocks. It is said that the Wittelsbach Dynasty was not very fond of the idea that the cheeky prince decided to become a racing driver. It's a lucky thing this was of no consequence to him, otherwise we would never have met.

Poldi is a real jewel. He takes his role as Patron of *dolphin aid* most seriously, and is distressed that his many representational duties and commitments don't leave him enough time to do all for our charity that he would wish to do. He sets himself aside from others in that he doesn't ask 'Where are the cameras' and thereupon takes a sick child in his arms, laughs to the camera, and then disappears.

The prince attends meetings of no special media interest, sits there for whole afternoons and talks with parents about their experiences. His sympathies and concerns are very real and come from the heart, and his conversation proves that he knows what he is talking about.

His wife, Her Royal Highness Princess Ursula von Bayern, and he also have a 'special needs' child.

After taking over the patronage of *dolphin aid* the two of them agreed to talk about their 'special daughter' in public. In the magazine *Bunte*, Poldi gave an interview of immense depth. Up until this point the couple had taken enormous care to protect their private lives, especially that of their children, from the invasion of the media.

Uncaring members of the press however made a meal out of this interview, even going so far as to print the headline *Princess Healed by Dolphins*. They unearthed, from the archives, a picture of the Princess Victoria of Sweden together with her brother prince Carl Phillip, the godson of Poldi, visiting a dolphinarium. This suspect action however brought a large donation into the hands of *dolphin aid* as His Royal Highness had, as an alternative, threatened legal proceedings against the aforementioned publisher.

In spite of this attack upon his private sphere, Poldi never has lost his enthusiasm to go out into the field for *dolphin aid*, for all the children and so also for Timmy. He has given the title 'patron' a completely new dimension. To know he is in our midst is a privilege.

In the meantime, for all personnel planning for *dolphin aid*, the quite normal madness had to continue. The number of families seeking help increases daily. It was quite clear that we would never collect enough donations to give assistance to all those seeking help, and that we needed to secure financial support.

We had to break out into new dimensions. We needed not only the private donors, whose hearts we had already reached, but a concept in order to win companies as sponsors.

With Dieter Hahn, the Personnel Director at LTU International Airways, I have a very special relationship. I accord him not only the greatest respect, I also like him very much. In the difficult times following Timmy's accident ,he never forgot to enquire about the condition of my son and signaled his will to help. It was Dieter Hahn who, in the end, gave me the advice to approach the head of the company, Dr Heinz Westen, with a view to deepening the bond between the airline and *dolphin aid*. He arranged in advance when and who had an appointment with Dr Westen, and two days later the secretary to the management called me to set a date for our meeting.

I was pretty nervous, armed with a concept which Michael and I had worked at in the course of many nights and put down on paper. Knowing that a top manager would have no more than ten minutes for me, I went to the appointment.

My meeting with Dr Westen lasted for more than two hours. After that I had to revise my notion that the atmosphere on the top management floors was a cool one. I returned home assured of help and full of admiration for this extraordinary man. The results of this meeting were clear to see for a long time in the media. Not only the airline, but the whole group followed the call of my son. Our modest search for help, which had begun with the unbureaucratic help of my colleagues, permanently reached new peaks.

New impulses have been given to *dolphin aid* by Marco Dadomo, the group head of communications and public relations and by Sabine Schwarzer the press chief of Meiers Weltreisen, who both became great promoters of our aims. The circle of people who enjoy a special place in my life is further increased by these two persons.

In the meantime we not only had 100 free flights at our disposal, not only too the donation of money for each booked passenger by the tour providers of the group, not only the visual message in the video program on board the flights, not only the invitation of the author in the on-board magazine to donate to our cause, but also through the collection of 'left-over' foreign currency on board all aircraft. With the help of all the staff, be it in the air or on the ground, at the lowest, the middle or in the upper management, *dolphin aid* has long got over its growing pains.

Following the example of our first sponsor, today many well known companies give their support and engage themselves for *dolphin aid*. The human fantasy knows no bounds when it comes to doing something to help the charity. For example the Munich Cart Palace held a series of go-cart races for the benefit of our charity, Kids Care and A Heart for Children (the charity of the *Bild* newspaper) are very strong partners, Nomi

Baumgartl produced a fantastic post-card calendar *dolphin aid*, phinware — based in Düsseldorf, sponsored flight tickets, Hapag Lloyd Cruises auctioned nautical maps on board their ships during cruises for the benefit of *dolphin aid*, DIS AG a personnel service company is certainly not mean when it comes to helping activities, and the company BMG in Cologne has persuaded some of the most famous names, and performers, in the musical world to produce a benefit CD for *dolphin aid*, and all of this makes it possible to be able to help even more children.

From the hurt a dream was born, and this dream took on form, and this form then became happiness, and from happiness a wish emerged, from this wish a vision, and the vision itself became a reality. This reality is *dolphin aid*.

From a modest charity, this great collection of dedicated persons, and I say that not without a great deal of pride, has grown to be an established and well-known organization, all in a short period of time.

The German pioneers made it financially possible to form the same foundation in America, for grief and pain know no borders. *Dolphin aid* in the USA was meant to be our, my, tribute to this wonderful country and to all those American 'special needs' children. The central point of all our activities is now in America, in Key Largo, Dr. Nathanson's Dolphin Human Therapy.

The first real friend I met whilst looking for an apartment was Veronica Cervera. This unbelievable woman, an engineer, beautiful but tough business lady, always the leader of every pack, one of the best girl friends possible, open, frank and direct in her speech, a loving family-manager with her Cuban soul, took me by the hand. She introduced me to the people I 'had to know'. She paved my way and made many things easier for me.

Veronica's husband Nickel Goesecke, Michael and I together were the founders of *dolphin aid* in America. Soon we found the necessary board members and formed a powerful team.

Christa Green from Northern Trust Bank became Vice-President; her significant 'other half' Stephen Cannon, President of Cybiz Partners, the attorney Alexander Reuss, the accountant Franz Carpraro, car sales and marketing expert Cathy Monceaux, 'India Silk' owner Madhu Mehta, Betty McManus, fertility expert Dr. Jürgen Eisermann, Pediatrician Dr. Ramon Guevara and not to forget the famous expert for rehabilitation Prof. Dr Bernard Brucker, are members of the board and the guarantee for inspirational decisions and operations in the sense of the articles of incorporation.

The success of *dolphin aid* has been made possible by the European media, and so I have to thank all those writers, photographers, presenters, interviewers, those who film and those who commentate. Without the indescribable presence in the media we would not have been able to help so many children, and the mention of dolphin therapy would only produce a shrug of the shoulders amongst the general public.

Our documentation within the media contains many reports of great sensitivity, many competent commentaries supported by understanding of the subject, and many simply wonderful stories. The radio interviews with deep feeling and the film documents about happy children and the hopes of their parents demonstrate our work in co operation with the therapy centers and have made *dolphin aid* an institution with an ever increasing presence in the public knowledge.

Each new thing, each win and success and each little battle won by *dolphin aid* have given these people reason to report about us, the team from *dolphin aid*. The way would have been far more difficult, and a far stonier one without their support, for the small private initiative we were at the beginning. And the sponsors would not have been so willing to jump into our boat.

The representatives of the media have allowed themselves to be carried by Timmy into what had been a closed world for them. Several of them have become addicted along the way. They want to see more laughing children's faces that yesterday were stone walls, and want to hear more from the child that learnt to speak his first word with Spunky & Marcy, want to hear once more the story of Timmy's laugh, that I already told so many times. And that's a wonderful thing.

One of the highlights to date in the love affair between the media and *dolphin aid* is the film *The Dolphin Wonder* aimed at bringing dolphin therapy home to a wide spectrum of the general public. I was allowed to work on the final script of the film. Following its viewing and various conferences a wonderful co-operation was born between the TV channel and airlines for the benefit of *dolphin aid*.

The consultations regarding the script were a completely new experience for me and I found it exciting to be a part of this.

When it was filmed in Key Largo I was able to get to know all the big and the small actors who were necessary in order to produce such a film. Kira is still today quite in love with the lead boy, Phillip, who for me, with his acting talent, carried the film. The story remained, in each scene, fictitious but drew from reality. At least so that one could say 'Yes it really could happen like that'.

The TV company organized a film gala, which was of course the premiere of the film, to honor us. Seven hundred people accepted the invitation of our patron and the director of programs. When I received the guest list at my hotel I asked my mother to make my excuses to the organizers. 'Please tell them I'm not well — I can't possibly make a speech in front of so many prominent people.' After page three of my speech, my nerves had calmed down and I think that I managed to get over to my listeners the message so near to my heart.

In the future too the journalists, producers, photographers and the presenters will play a big part in the success of *dolphin aid*. We can only hope that it will continue this way in America, and possibly all over the world. Then only with the help of the representatives of the media can we find financial support to realize the dream of a pure therapy and research center. And this with the best possible natural environment for the dolphins and a better future for so many children who especially need our help.

The present

It took a long time before I was really in a suitable state to tell this story. The memories had damaged the deepest parts of my soul.

It didn't occur to me, at first, what was happening to me during the nights while I was working to put my thoughts on paper.

With the same urge which had driven me to found *dolphin aid*, I decided to write Timmy's story, quite certain in the knowledge that at all times and with each line I wrote, somewhere in the world a mother, or father or a whole family may find themselves at that exact time in the glare of fluorescent lighting, and the horrid reality of some Intensive Care Unit. That they may have to endure all that which I had experienced, the fear, the despair, being as if paralyzed, the hurt that cripples every fibre of your body, and with the hope to awake sometime from the nightmare.

I wanted to help others to master their own paths, by passing on my experiences. I wanted to shout out loud 'Look here, don't just cry, — you will be able to manage it', the way that Timmy has managed it, and how I too have learned to manage it; you will learn again to laugh, and at some point again have that feeling that the sun is shining, even though it may never be so warm again.

And when I began to reminisce about Timmy's accident, and to scratch about in those innermost parts of my secret soul, looking for the fragments that I only knew because they had been told to me, and began to commit to paper those things that I thought I had forgotten, I found myself shaken with vomiting cramps, bent over the toilet again.

At first I thought I had eaten something which had not agreed with me. When the same thing happened the following night, I gave the blame to the entire pack of cigarettes which I had smoked, whilst writing, within the space of two hours, between two and four in the morning.

Even on the third night I had not the foggiest idea what was happening to me and this time blamed the half bottle of wine with which I had made myself comfortable at the computer in those sleepy hours.

The following morning it hit me like a bolt of lightning. Neither on the first or on the following nights did my sickness have anything to do with any of the reasons I had blamed.

It was much worse than this: I had begun to 'sick-up' and 'spit out'; at first without comprehending, and later with an all too clear knowledge. I had begun, at last, to sort things out in my heart and soul. I had slowly started to work on my mourning, which in the past years I had not allowed to happen, because I did not want to allow it to happen, and either consciously or deep in my mind I believed that any breakdown or weakness on my part may, in the worst case, have had a fatal consequence for Timmy.

My helplessness, which I hid away behind the seemingly endless activity, and the creeping feeling of total solitude inside of me, was openly revealed there on the desk in front of me. Through my own energy I was now suddenly forced to think about my exact emotional state of mind, with no chance of covering it over again in a frenzied activity.

Naturally I said to myself 'You don't really want to write this book — what the hell for?', at the beginning. After a while I gazed lovingly at my abandoned writing desk and the story began to take form in my thoughts. In day dreams I wrote chapter after chapter, without actually putting anything down on paper. And I loved this book, that no one but myself could read. It was my life, and that of my children and a few other people, who, in the course of all the troubles, had become, for me, irreplaceable.

Almost automatically, certainly not deliberately I began to elucidate myself, my role as daughter, mother,

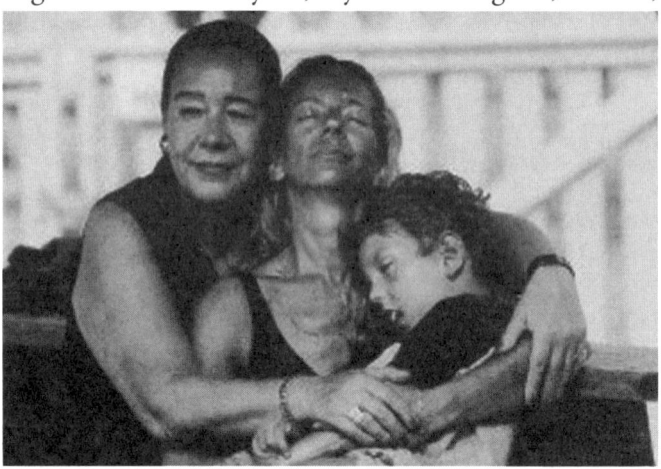

Kindred spirits — three generations

life-partner, ex-wife and as a friend. That which I discovered sometimes led me to laugh about myself. I had certainly changed in the last few years. The main reason for this was Timmy, and also Kira. Naturally I still possess the same bad habits, weaknesses, the same strengths and the same understanding of friendship, of ethics, of morals and faithfulness, from social commitment and also from love. But the number of people who are now in a position to hurt me has reduced drastically.

For the very first time in my life then I began to like myself — for example as a daughter.

Most certainly I was for my mother what the Americans call 'a pain in the butt'. My mother is a wonderful person and an outstanding personality, but as a mother I found her awful. I have always loved her but I always felt there was something missing — 'I missed the chocolate pudding for dessert'. She was my friend and I her mirror reflection, and for this reason she had sometimes hated me as much as I hated her. Rather after the saying 'One day you wake up look into the mirror — and there grinning back at you is the image of your mother'.

For more than thirty years I had tried every trick in the book to gain her attention and approval. Without success. In my family all are born with that song on their lips *I'm a little king*.

And today? My heart warms when I think of my mother. I am thankful to her that she had made me what I am today, that she brought me up giving me the ability to weather, for almost more than seven years now, the storm without ever having given up, that she enriched my heart and my soul with values, for whose continuation in this world I worry, and which I definitely want to pass on to my children. And I am thankful that my parental home furnished me with the confidence which enables me, with a natural openness, to confront everyone.

After all the upsets of a classic mother and daughter drama and conflict we now have the respect for each other of two grown-up women who have absolutely nothing to hide from one another. We have never before had the wish to spend as much time together as possible.

And she is the best grandmother in the world, without any of the apron clichés. She reads aloud fairy stories, full of energy, and knows all the words to the children's songs of my childhood. And today she can even make chocolate pudding. Only, not for me.

Grandmothers appear to be mothers who have been given a second chance. At some stage I am sure that my children will pack their bags with the wish 'We're moving in with granny!'. And that's life.

And what kind of a mother am I myself? How am I, disregarding Tim's conditon, as a mother? In this question I must be careful not to be self-satisfied. But I find myself super.

Children are the last true absolute adventure. I found my children to be an enrichment to my life from the very first day. Children are the true teachers, their natural unbending openness, their natural charm, their eye for that which is really important, who register the smallest vibrations, their undamaged upright stature and their thirst for knowledge, their spirit of investigation and their life in the 'here and now' — all that brightens everyday life. This energy-consuming realization can be, in the daily happenings with one another, also very wearing, especially when my children, with painful clarity, expose my own weaknesses and at the slightest failure bore their little fingers into the wound. 'You may not say shit', intoned Kira. 'I don't really like this food', 'But yesterday you promised', 'You've also left your things lying on the floor in the bathroom'. There's nothing worse in the world than being caught red-handed. And also Timmy, mostly speechless at present, still leaves no doubt about the times he thinks his mother has messed things up.

But the children forgive me quickly, then they know that I drive happily to the kindergarten, to tennis, to ballet, or to therapy A, B, C, and to doctor X, Y, Z. Whenever they want to they can sleep 'In the big bed'. Apart from all this I'm good at French fries, make a great spaghetti, can look after playmates, and the way to the zoo, the circus, to the fair or to the fairytale woods I know like the back of my hand. When I look at our lives from all sides, I come to the decision that, although sometimes I shout the place down, in the end I can, with peace of mind, draw the conclusion that I am a dependable, self critical and jolly companion who encourages their personal skills but who also respects their unique personalities.

And that most likely, at the end of the day, I am sure that I need them more than they need me — and besides that I make good chocolate pudding. The verdict as to my role as an ex-wife would be less positive, either looked at from the one side or the other.

Looking at it realistically I had every reason to heap hate for evermore upon my husband. If I had started to write this book earlier I would probably go down into the annals in doubtful writing history. I wanted to tell the whole world what my husband had done to me and my children, from my point of view, with his shallow emotions, lack of responsibility and his phlegmatic attitude. And now? Time has mellowed me.

Our marriage was really over, but a further year we continued to live together and deliver scenes which would make a good film. On reflection I'm very pleased that in our elegant hallway there hung no chandelier, as in the movie *War of the Roses*.

After this followed a time of cold distance, each always ready to jump, in a permanent fighting spirit. The longer we were separated the clearer I could see our relationship. If I had had to express, at the time of our parting, the responsibility as a percentage, I would have assessed my part at a maximum of 30%. But in the course of time and a clear head, looking at things from a distance, the picture changes. Today it's simply just a few particular happenings that stick in my mind.

I have found many excuses with which to give my husband the absolution for his failings. He was too young, he wasn't mature enough, he suffered from having a dominant father who was a wonderful man with a lot of heart, but always careful to keep all the strings in his hands. Sometimes I ask myself today who it was I was married to.

Just like a little mouse I tried to set myself against the opinions from outside, said 'No, no, no', loud and clear — and then in a small voice conceded 'Yes' instead of sticking with my point of view, and by the first 'No'. My own fault.

The sweet disposition of my father-in-law who wished for a constant line of caring dependence, without any loopholes within the family, had regretfully not passed this on to his eldest son. Therefore, behind the scenes we had constant battles in which I was less of a mouse and more a bitch. My poor husband. Even today he has certainly still not understood why I fought against this dependency with every fibre of my body, and why I did not want my father-in-law to have the last word regarding decisions to be made for my family.

He had grown up with this and therefore was not able to understand my strong will for independence to make the decisions concerning my family ourselves.

Besides I must say that, from today's view, after a given point I had forgotten that I was not only a mother but also a wife and not just part of a parent's partnership. With a never ending desire for discussion I bombarded my husband with speeches loaded with criticism about his behavior within the family, I couldn't see that he was as if paralyzed after Timmy's accident. I went into action, he did not.

I have suffered, while feeling permanently left alone by him, without realizing that he was not mature enough for the job. For the ways and means he tried to come to terms with the situation, I loathed him.

The single accusation which we would both have to admit was possibly that we didn't try everything to save our relationship. We were unable to free ourselves from the current of aggression and at some stage I decided to invest the energy that I still had in my children instead of on the battlefield of my marriage.

The best thing about this bitter experience is that in spite of wounds which have hardly healed I can say: 'I left my husband although I still loved him, and a part of me will always love him, also because he is the father of my children, for whose existence I am thankful. And because I do well to remember I married him out of total conviction.'

Without a doubt my patience of today, and the diplomacy needed to cope with a partnership, which I have learnt the hard way, would have helped me to save my marriage, but perhaps we were not mature enough.

From his point of view I am certainly, as ever, his 'trouble and strife' his mobile bad conscience, the one who detects every lie and for whom he can't 'pull the wool over her eyes'. I can live with that. Maybe we shall meet again one day in an old people's home and remember together that we got married purely out of love. But until then it's OK the way it is. What's the saying? 'Maybe one day we can become good friends.'

To analyze my role as a life partner is much more difficult — most likely because it's quite clear to me how hard it is to live with me. I have tried naturally in the past few years to integrate the knowledge gained from the past to flow into my relationship with Michael, who out of being a trusted person and my best friend, has become my life partner. But it was he who gave me the opportunity to develop further. Especially in the daily intimacies within which I have learned much from him.

He has taught me to live the theory that every medal has two sides.

But still, now and then, I come close to my limits, have a tendency to impatience and still expect my partner to react the way I want him to.

But in our relationship there are two chiefs and no Indians, and in daily life just this can sometimes cause problems. Apart from this I must say that it appears to me, without meaning to be a militant feminist, that men quite simply have a reduced understanding of things. I am sure that I am far away from being an emancipate: I simply enjoy too much being a woman. I prefer to go through a door which is held open for me rather than to risk getting it in the face from the gentleman in front of me. I hate every form of degrading bad manners and love polished behavior. I am not the home-baked type, and as 'just a housewife' would drive any man crazy, cleaning the whole day just for something to do.

I am a very creative person and constantly have new ideas, and so that has to be done straight away. I am far too quick in my thoughts, I'm just talking about one thing and in my mind at the same time I have already passed on to the next — and before he knows where I am, my partner in conversation is not sure if I'm still quite sane.

So obviously I am not really the oasis of peace in a stressed manager's life, but Michael enjoys my comments on his business plans. Sometimes, though, when they do not agree with his concept, it can be pretty exhausting.

Depending on his mood, he will sometimes discuss with me the controversy, but in secret probably thinks of the times past when his companions just simply stood back and admired him. I admire him too, naturally, but not quite so often!

I can quite easily go shopping without a list, can book flights, put my signature to contracts and fill out my voting form by myself, I can fill my car with petrol and call the man to repair the washing machine. And I say so sometimes — and that pretty loudly.

What about our relationship? What makes it such a special one?

Why does a clear-thinking man take on a woman of changeable moods, who is not always easy to handle — one with two children and one of those a 'Special needs' child?

To start with, our life is never boring. We always have something to tell one another. We need no other company. We have the same taste in many things, and in others quite different. Who cares! Added to this, Michael is the best father that my children could ever wish for, and for that reason I love him most especially.

Naturally he has his quirks which are hard to cope with. As a 'Leo' he has to be admired and cheered on, and when not — be careful!

I have advanced to a fairly competent cheer-leader in order, if only from time to time, to satisfy this need.

In spite of all the pressures from outside, the lack of time together alone and a completely private sphere, the missing honeymoon, and the unfulfilled dreams of times 'just for us two', we have a nice time together. Sometimes there's a row or two, but that's healthy and anyway it clears the air.

Without him I would not be the person I am today. Without him my children would not be able to define, or even spell, the word father. Without him many little miracles would not have been possible, because I had not been able to see them. And I hope I will never have to say 'Without him...'

There are no people who would say 'Mrs Kuhnert, 'Kiki'. Oh well, you know she's OK' — and this defines my part of friendship quite simply. There are only people who say 'super' or 'catastrophe', and so it's impossible for the 'maybe' people to feel well in my surroundings. It's either yes or no.

How much I've changed in the past years is mirrored in the circle of friends I have. I have to thank Timmy that today the people I am surrounded by can reach clear verdicts. Remarkable, and a compliment, is that companions of old days, who had difficulty getting on with me following the separation of 'the pair' are now sometimes found sitting on my sofa these days and are really pleased that the bond of old times has been retied. That is a sign of maturity, that two sides can approach one another because they have understood the point of view of the other and were not too shy to admit mistakes, even if this is sometimes without words.

For me friendship is something of great value. Betrayal, disloyalty and lies are things, which in my opinion, can only lead to the end of friendship.

But I have also learnt that I can't push my point of view down the throats of my friends.

By the same token where I have become more tolerant and less demanding on one hand, on the other I have become, deep inside me, without compromise regarding my peace of mind and anything which would damage that — mine or my little family's world.

I hope I am excused for saying so, but the naked truth is that the number of people, who may 'Kiss my Ass', naturally increases daily.

In my little world I no longer tolerate people who just live to create intrigues or who are filled with jealousy for what ever, therefore disturbing our circle and are of no use to anyone, except to cause trouble. Instead of the egoists, the ignorant and the psychopaths of this world, I prefer dreamers, visionaries and the slightly mad who have depth to their character, who maybe give food for thought in their fantasies, and with whom I can have a decent conversation and laugh heartily. In view of my own failings, my friends can also 'put their foot in it' but also be assured of my complete support when they fail doing things in which they truly believe.

Isn't it that what makes a friendship, being there for each other in any situation? Even though this is what I have not experienced much of, I'm still quite certain that it pays to believe it.

One of my new friends, funnily enough, the ex-husband of the present life companion of my ex-husband, who lives together with the godmother of my daughter, recently quite threw me 'I wouldn't take all the money in the world to change places with you — but I would give all the money in the world to be like you'. At this I cried.

The darker side

In spite of all efforts to put aside all the terrible things to do with Timmy's accident I have been forced during the past, now more than seven years, nevertheless to face up to and cope with them.

The avalanche of legal steps was set in motion by the family lawyers without my instigation. My point of view was quite definite. Timmy would not return to health through any legal verdict and so I found every court appointment to be just another burden. I was against all this — not over and over again to have to relive the tortuous pain that accompanies me permanently anyway.

Little by little I was forced to learn what it meant to be responsible for a 'special needs' child, the financial sacrifices which had to be made in order to be able to give him the best possible care. At some stage I found that I was not even properly medically insured and so I had to ensure that my own insurance and that of my children was secured, and that costs a hell of a lot of money every month.

Without any complaints I gave up my career — it was the only way possible to get my life organized. That meant too that I was totally without any income. Because of my economic problems, begging from the family and the permanent financial pressures, I slowly sharpened my decision to make the court case against the owner of the restaurant where we had held Kira's christening. In the end I wanted justice to be given its proper place.

The mere existence of this no-longer used swimming pool, its location and its condition, I was to learn later, had, in the local golf club, often been the issue of many heated discussions at members' meetings. They were afraid that after parties and celebrations, with alcohol, people leaving the function room, a barn, could fall into this pool without being noticed and drown.

What an irony of fate that of all people my son should be the one. Forty hours after his tragic accident, he was responsible for the destruction of the scene of the accident, on order of the authorities and with the help of a bulldozer. If only before ... if, if, if ... And it was this damn thing that was, for Timmy, destiny. My son was, as I read in the court records almost four years after the catastrophe, drowned in even less than one and a half foot of stagnant water. A swimming pool, no longer in use, behind some bushes and with no fencing or protection, a matter of some 15 metres from the terrace of the public restaurant where I was myself — the place where all were gathered who were the stars in the heaven of his little life.

Did I not give proper supervision? For, as we left the church, an argument had almost broken out because my parents-in-law wanted to take Timmy in their convertible Mercedes to the golf club and the car had no child's seat and I was frightened that he, sitting strapped on the jump seat at the back, could come to harm. If only I had answered this anxiety instead of 'for the sake of peace' and wanting to avoid any family quarrel which would possibly have spoilt Kira's christening, said to myself that in those few metres drive all would be well — if I would have rushed off home with two healthy children and left behind me the invited and astonished guests... How many times since then have I wished that I had had one of my famous temperamental outbreaks. If only...

Have I loaded guilt upon myself because, just for a few minutes, I wanted a moment to myself, and left my child in the care of the people who were, anyway, most important in his life, with the safe feeling that he was cosseted in a cocoon of love, warmth and gentleness, probably being passed from one lap to another?

In the end the feeling would remain that I should not, even for this short moment, have left him alone, and been at his side as I always was. But I was tied up with the happenings only a few metres away, through the open door, and yet light years away.

Can I today renounce the charge that I had failed in my responsibility, with a clear conscience?

Yes I can — basically, morally, ethically and philosophically! And for more than seven years I have had to prove that in front of the court. How many long hours must I spend reading the nerve-killing statements of evidence. I still am absolutely perplexed at the efforts of the other side to divert all responsibility from themselves and to play for time, because it's a question of money!

The opposition has, right up to this date, never troubled itself to ask about the condition of my child, or to express their regrets at what happened, nor have they ever once offered any help. Instead there is the loaded atmosphere of a case still in progress. The nerves of a mother and her psychological condition are merely reduced to things of no consequence — a by-product.

A quite unbelievable thing happened when the report was compiled in order to estimate the life expectancy of my son, to be able to calculate a pension, upon which he could live. The suspicious assessor was absolutely astonished when I insisted upon taking my son out of the room before his estimated date of death should be announced. Quite clearly he could not imagine how one could inflict psychological damage on such an uncommunicative 'piece of meat'. I would recommend most earnestly that the mentioned professor read the book *Diving Bell and Butterflies* in which a person in a 'locked-in syndrome' still manages to communicate his feelings by the blinking of an eye. Perhaps the contents of the book may help to increase his field of imagination.

During the last court session it was finally over with my discipline and my self castigation. After three hours of court session my patience was at an end and I shouted at one of the witnesses. The judge did not even warn me to control myself. When I apologized for my outbreak the judge turned to the witness, and said 'We all have all the understanding in the world, don't we?'.

It was the closing day of the court hearing, at least that of the High Court. Our lawyer, who appeared to be exactly the right man for the job, was sure that everything had gone well. He had taken care of us well over the years, and as the judge offered a compromise, I stood there absolutely without an idea, and not in any state to make a decision anyway. Our lawyer said that we owed it to Timmy to go through with things to the bitter end. That calmed me a little and gave me impetus.

The next step will be to the Federal Court of Law. I fear I will not be spared this.

Joy

My Mother, with tears in her eyes, often told me about her pain, of her worries about me, her only child and her sorrow due to Timmy's sad condition.

Filled with bitterness, she speaks at these moments about how much it weighs down upon her that my life has taken this direction — from all the hopes and wishes which she had for me at my birth, from all her efforts to make my path a happy and, wherever possible, an easy one — her hopes, that, at the end of our story, great joy and happiness should wait for me and my children.

Not very long ago we had 'one of those' conversations and, as we spoke I recognized something wonderful, I noticed it myself only as I listened to my own words, trying to reduce her fears and bitterness.

I am happy! I am really filled with Joy.

Even in spite of the daily fights and the persistent worries, I have truly become a deeply satisfied person. My son has shown me so much. And he has taught me what happiness really means. Not only has he sharpened my senses and my emotions but has also opened them. He has taught me a wonderful modesty. And he has shown me to enjoy intensively the happy moments and to use them as a source of energy for the next drama, for the next challenge.

Timmy has made it possible for me to accept defeats, for tomorrow is another day. And most important of all he has taught me to live in the 'here and now'. Not in the past nor in the future, but today.

For good or bad, who knows what tomorrow will bring? And yesterday — that really seems to be ages ago.

I find today that, to be taken notice of for whatever reason at all, be it love, thankfulness, or from respect or recognition, is a great and special privilege.

I know now what happiness is. The little miracles every day. Also the failures and disappointments are part of it — for only those who have tasted bitter wine can appreciate the sparkling taste of champagne. And when you have learnt this, then even the cheapest bottle from the supermarket is fine.

Therefore I can smile at my mother, with a clear conscience and say 'I am happy, quite independently from all other outside influences, I, for myself, am really happy'.

On those mornings when my daughter, out of sheer joy and excitement, wakes me with 'Mami, Mami you must come and see the sunrise' then I know it will be a good day. I know in these moments that Kira is happy because I have been able to show her to see the beauty of the sunrise.

Then I know what happiness is.

When I think that in all the bad times I had my family by my side, especially my big uncle Volker, who could not reduce my troubles, but who helped me financially wherever he could so that I, at least sometimes, was released from the problems of naked survival — my family who assumed one of the most important roles in my life when things were at their very worst. And when I look into the deepest parts of my soul and sense my thankfulness, then I know what happiness is.

When I think of my father, who I have now only truly found, and experience the gentle understanding love which he has for me, then I know what happiness is.

When I think of that handful of people whom I thought I had lost along my stony path following Tim's accident, and have found again, then I know what happiness is.

When I think what has become of *dolphin aid*, in the clear knowledge that this organization brings sunshine into the lives of 'special needs' children, and that the members of the large *dolphin aid* family feel themselves fortunate that no one asks 'What have you cried about today?'. Also then I know what happiness is.

When I remember all the people I have met along my path, who lightened my spirit and reached my soul, and went part of the way with me. Then I know what happiness is.

When I think of all those who allowed themselves to be inspired by Timmy and who followed the call of his soul to help not only him but also other hopeless children, then I know what happiness is.

When I feel that safe, certain, Mother love with which I am bound to my children, and how important we are to one another, when the natural symbiosis of our little family system becomes visible and perceptible, and when I know that I will always love both my children exactly the way they are, to follow them with no 'ifs' and 'buts' in all stages of their possible development, then I know what happiness is.

When I hold my partner's hand, while trying to find my way through seemingly impossible chaos, and I feel his love reach me to give me courage, when he, nearly on the point of a nervous breakdown, forgives me for hurting him, and then wraps me in his arms, and when at night I hear his breath and know that I am not alone, because he shares with me all the burdens the best he can. Then, especially then, I know what happiness is.

And when, last of all, I imagine that Timmy one day, right at the end of this story, has, in front of him, a fully independent happy life to live, one in which he can always rely on the love of his sister. When this time comes, I am sure that the happiness will be so overwhelming that I will not be able to comprehend, and will spend my life just floating. The most important people will say to me on this day, 'Kiki, could you come back down to earth from up there for a moment?' because then, at last, I would know exactly what happiness is.

A journey through time

Dolphin Human Therapy is certainly still the main reason for our trips to Florida, but in the course of the years we have not only found a 'home from home' in Miami but also enlarged the therapy team surrounding Timmy, with highly qualified specialists. Professor Bernard Brucker, director of the 'Biofeedback-Laboratory' at the University of Miami Jackson Memorial Hospital, has become an irreplaceable help for Tim. The scientist and doctor won me over from the very first second by his manner.

The first time he assessed Tim, in the course of a session lasting several hours, he greeted Barbara, whom I had brought along for support, and me with friendliness, but was quite short. He took a chair and sat himself down in front of Tim and then proceeded for well over an hour to explain to him, while holding his head gently in his hands, all about neuro-muscular bio-feedback, what it was all about, what could be recorded on the computer and how this would be done; what this treatment would mean for Tim and also what aims, he, Dr Brucker, had for him.

My son was as fascinated as Barbara and myself. He listened to the professor the whole time, fully taken in, and began to give vocal answers in his own language.

After more than an hour Professor Brucker ended his descriptions with the words, 'And what do you think Timmy? Has your mother any further questions?'.

Timmy blossomed visibly, naturally his mother had no further questions, all was a matter for the two men now.

After Timmy had followed all the instructions of the American doctor, almost without any delay between question and carrying out the request, and I had followed, or at least tried to follow, I learnt for the first time in my life, to love a computer.

With the help of electrodes fixed to his back, Timmy spoke to us, through this electronic machine. Naturally he didn't speak in words but in the terms of values assessed on the screen, he was able to show that he had understood every single word of the English speaking professor and not only that he had understood and comprehended but also that he had immediately tried to put the words into actions.

Now we knew that his limits were purely physical, that his ears heard all and transmitted this to his little head which was functioning too, and the brain that had been declared as irreparably damaged began to sort out and to pass on the information. We learnt that this is where the problems began, at the nerve channels to the individual parts of the body.

I cried an awful lot. Barbara was 'all-in', her professional worldly concept of things in conjunction with Timmy had sometimes wobbled anyhow, but now we both stood in front of the clinic, cigarette in hand, and trembling — and starting again and again to laugh and cry — making it clear to Timmy how immensely proud of him we were.

I had always been right. I wasn't quite mad. Timmy understood every word! — and that also in English!

All the time I had been certain that Timmy's understanding of language was completely bi-lingual, but out of fear of being delivered into a funny farm I had never told anyone. They wouldn't have believed me anyway.

Carried away in this mood of freedom and at the same time in the middle of preparing for our first American Christmas, I received a fax from Dr Ibach, requesting that I visit him in Remscheid. He asked that I speak with him immediately upon my return to Germany.

As the result of various reports about dolphin therapy he had received requests from all sides, and it was generally known that he was the doctor who, on that fateful day of Timmy's accident, had treated him.

Happily I followed his request. It was his words about my child on that dreadful day which in the long and endless after, had given me courage in my times of deepest despair. 'There's a 95% chance ... for the other 5% we are on the outside looking in, we can't tell'. Since then I had been searching for the 95%, for there must have been something which made him believe that Timmy would survive this trauma, retaining no permanent damage.

It was therefore that I drove on a grey January morning to Remscheid and looked forward to seeing this sensitive doctor again. Just before turning into the road where the hospital was, I began to tremble. I shook that much that I was hardly able to drive on. My teeth chattered although I was not cold. Tears coursed over my cheeks and I lost control of both my nerves and my body.

What a silly fool I was. I had never for one minute or even one second thought about what it would mean to me to return to the clinic for the first time after years.

How clever, or how strong did I think I was?

Completely taken aback at my reaction I entered the clinic, trembling still. The smell, which truly is different in every hospital, almost made me be sick. As if in a dream I told the secretary who I was and what I wanted. I felt as if I was being powered by remote-control.

Dr Ibach and I spoke for much longer than was planned. He wanted to know everything about Timmy, so that I had to call home in the meantime to make sure that everything was in order.

As if in a trance I decided to visit the Intensive Care Ward. I wanted to see again the sisters, and I wanted, as I had done so many times in my nightmares, to experience, once again, the way it was.

The return trip home turned into a never ending journey back into the past. One more time everything passed before my eyes, as if in a film.

The moment they asked me 'Is Timmy with you? — the search in sheer panic — the sight, as they rescued my son — my scream — the never ending efforts to bring him back to life, the rescue helicopter, the same nightmare I keep meeting these days — the one that is hiding behind some bush on the highway, waiting to shock me.

And as if one more time it was reality, he flies away from me in this movie.

And again I have this death wish — I can't go on. Timmy has drowned, I smell the Intensive Care Unit, as if I was still there, hear the voice of my son calling to me, as it happened to me in this particular night after the accident. I relive the endless yearning for my daughter, my baby, that I had not been allowed to give in to for months. I rock in the chair in which I spent weeks on end at Timmy's bedside, see the images of doctors, good and bad, friendly and less friendly, whose names I have long since forgotten.

I see the visitors to the hospitals, their incomprehension and their tears, the nursing sisters, who were pleased that I could at last cry, those who cared for Timmy, I fly to Rome with my children — and all this within the space of a few minutes.

I see healers and quacks, feel hope and despair in the same measure as in the moments when they were reality. I see my children growing up, feel the pain in my heart, when Kira invents the same words as Timmy, experience the day when Kira overtakes Timmy and there are no more comparisons possible, because Timmy's natural further development ended that same day.

I drive along the road to therapy, there and back, keep guard on all of those nights of broken sleep that happened for years, and I worry about Kira's undamaged development, speak to specialists, and notice that my energy seems to be coming to an end, only to recover almost immediately and almost out of spite, to fight the next fight.

Within seconds I fly back and forth to America, dolphins swim through my thoughts, therapists smile at me, the sun warms my skin ...

With this feeling of warmth I recall a story that someone once told me.

Especially for my friend Biggi Feldmann I would like to write this story down. There is a very deep bond between us for she, too, has a 'special needs' child.

Phillip was born one year before Timmy. She had advised me to have an amniocentesis test. She was one of those women who, before the birth of her child, I would never have imagined being capable of caring for a 'special needs' child. Without her, there would have been many names I never heard, lots of questions I would never have asked, and many paths I would never have found. Timmy would not even have that damn handicapped identity card if it were not for her. I want to dedicate this story especially to her:

God hovered above the Earth and chose with great care and thought his instruments for the protection of the species.

He observed everything carefully and dictated to his angels from his internal propagation book.

'Betty Miller, daughter, guardian angel Matthew; Ivy Smith, son, guardian angel Gabriel; Carol King, son, guardian angel? Give her Jonathan, he's used to swearing.

At the end he dictated to an angel a name to write down, and said with a smile, 'I'll give her a handicapped child'.

The angel is astonished. 'Why have you chosen her God? She's so happy.'

'That's exactly why', God said, and continued to smile. 'How can I give a sick child to a mother who can't laugh? That would be cruel.'

'She doesn't have much patience either', the angel said.

'I don't want her to have patience. Otherwise she will drown in a sea of sadness and self pity. When the first pain and shock have passed, she will pick herself up and get on with things flawlessly. I watched her today. She has the right feeling of independence and self confidence. And that, alas, is very rare in mothers, but absolutely necessary. Listen to me — the child that I give her will live in another, in its own world. She must encourage it, and bring it so far that it lives in her world. That won't be easy.'

'But Lord', said the angel, 'as far as I can see she doesn't even believe in you'.

And God grinned to himself.

'That doesn't matter. Ill take care of that. Yes, yes, I think that she will be very capable. She is egoist enough.'

The angel gasped for breath: — 'Egoist? Is that really something good?'

God answered with a yes. 'When she doesn't sometimes distance herself from the child, she will not survive the burden, and it will be hard for her anyway, to cope with everything. It's exactly this woman to whom I will give a child that is not perfect. She doesn't know it, but she is really someone to be jealous of. She will never take a spoken word for granted, not a single step as something everyday and normal. When her child says Mama, for the first time, it will be clear to her that this is a miracle that she is experiencing. When she describes to her blind child a tree or a sunset, she will see these things as only a few see my creations. I will make it possible for her to recognize everything which I recognize. Cruelty, prejudice, ignorance. I will allow her to rise above these things. She will never be alone. Every day of her life, every minute. Because she does my work as surely as if she were sitting next to me.'

Still the tears course over my cheeks and I taste their saltiness. We have managed to come so far, Timmy has managed it. We will not give in even when the most horrid of times becomes reality again. And together we shall continue to manage.

It has taken a long time to get over the result of this needless, yet planned visit. I was too naive in the estimation of my own emotional state, or to put it better, I hadn't thought properly about it at all. What was positive in this experience was that I was able to see Timmy from a distance, and to analyze his development, as far as a mother can, objectively.

From the German guidelines, diagnoses and its accompanying language, Timmy is still a 'multiply handicapped child' who cannot manage the daily things alone and therefore is dependent upon 24 hour a day care.

I hate this description, while all the little steps of progress, all the victories that we have achieved together with much effort are put depressingly into question. Then Timmy is, above all, a happy child and also well-balanced. He has understood. He knows too that we have understood.

He and I communicate most successfully. He loves it when my language drifts away from that expected of a lady, grins sweetly when I swear again, hoping that Kira will not hear. And he turns his head towards me with the most enchanting smile when I ask him for a kiss. The flirt.

We are a team. Everything that has to be done, is bound up with a higher scale of difficulty. But we're together and when not taking three steps backwards, we set off together continually forward.

If we had ever lost the energy or the courage, or relied upon that which others said, if we would never have met the dolphins, and we would not have met, almost miraculously, in the depths of each deep, dark valley, wonderful people, Timmy would be lying in a care bed somewhere, breathing on a machine, being fed through a tube, choking and dribbling. And possibly he would be as clear in his head as he is now, and his suffering would be unbearable, but no-one would know it.

And through everything I have learnt, in all that I know and sense, I stick to the American description of 'special needs' children. My son is exactly that, a child with special needs. No more and no less ...

Today is Yesterday's Future

What a shame. Everything has to come to an end and this book must come to a close. But really it could be a *Never Ending Story.*

Every single day new and exciting things happen. That which others watch on TV happens to me almost on a daily basis. But I cannot just go on writing, writing, writing, enough for another book! Already today Kira complained 'All the time you just write!'. Of course that's not true.

From the many, many hours completely immersed in this world of writing, she has only experienced a very small part. For the daily 'madness' in my life leaves me very little time during daylight hours for literary 'spouting'.

'Out of the chaos a voice spoke to me "Laugh and be happy, it could be even worse". And I laughed and was happy – and it came even worse!!!!'

And to think I had always dreamed of .... residing in a rose garden, in delightful peace, with silken scarf wound around my throat, sipping now and again on a glass of champagne (merely to wet my lips), a whisper of classical music in the background, the gentle chatter of birdsong completing the whole scene tastefully.

Unfortunately it was not to be. As soon as I thought that I had an hour for myself, in order to compose at least a few sentences on paper, for this purpose I would retire to my office, which in the daytime was also the diaper-station for Timmy, because of the stairs. I would just close the door, and it would fly open again. 'Listen Mami, when are we going again to Fritzi's?'. 'Listen Mami, when is Grandma coming?'.

Or the phone would ring – it does so pretty much non-stop anyway, or there is a duet between the home line and the cell phone. Or Piroschka, or Lisa, - 'Excuse me, where can I find ...'.

Nobody seems to have understanding for a poor and damaged literary nervous system. Even in the really creative moments no one seemed to have any consideration. It was all the same to them whether I had a brilliant idea, or whether I may have even been able to have one!

Naturally my creative heart was bitten to the core by the incessant chattering of those favourite people around me, who had no idea that to write a portion of world literature one needs a quiet and inspiring surrounding.

I had to create my masterpiece alone.

And so I tried the more brittle touch. Like a Diva, you could say. I took as my models Hollywood stars, and tried simply to throw my head back, stopped short however at throwing the silver – and ended up more as a parody.

Nevertheless I thought that I could still arouse the necessary guilty feelings. They would be the ones responsible when the entire world was not enriched by my thoughts. It didn't help!!

In the end they began a conspiracy together. The opinion was united — I was just bad-tempered. 'Mami is not in a good mood!' What a laugh!!

And so I am a little proud that I was able to get it done — and to have that itching-in-the-fingers feeling go, along with the pain in my neck from sitting long hours at the computer in a pose which is not orthopaedically recommended.

And then in 1999 was the day when I first saw the book, MY BOOK, on the shelves of the book stores.

What happened then was extremely overwhelming in many ways. I was prepared for TV and Newspaper interviews. Also I expected some letters from parents with special needs children, with questions about Dolphin Human Therapy. I was in no way prepared for what actually happened. Tons of letters arrived in my mailbox, hundreds every day.

Some letters were from families with similar destinies. There were letters from husbands, who reduced their working load, changed their habits and started to spend more time with their wife and kids, letters from people who were well off but had always something to complain about although living healthy lives and with no financial worries, letters from Kids and from Grandmas. They mainly thanked me for showing them very clearly how valuable life is and how fragile our happiness is at any time.

I remember one very special letter that I would like to share with you. A middle-aged gentleman wrote the following: '… you and your story have changed my life. Whenever I feel a little down and start to feel pity for myself I only have to remember your story and what you went through and then I realize that whatever I have to experience in my daily life, whatever I think is a problem — it is really nothing compared with what you have experienced. And therefore looking at things that made me angry before or sad or nervous, today I can smile and I realize how well off I am — at any time. Actually I am more happy and even thankful for some of the problems that I have. Thank you for that.'

Also my book became a practical help for people who are in difficult situations. Still many questions were being asked. Looking back over the response to my book in the last 2 years there are mainly three questions asked by readers from many different countries and I have decided that the answers to those should be in the first English edition of this book:-

1. How is Timmy today and what has happened since I first wrote our story down on paper?
2. How did I manage to see this through?
3. What exactly is Dolphin Human Therapy and how does it work?

How is Timmy?

From my personal point of view the most important news is that Timmy is 'doing great'. He has grown tremendously, and is getting very heavy! Thank goodness I have, amongst my friends, an Olympic weight lifter who gave me advice on carrying techniques, so at least I don't have back pains. I am still certain that it is only a question of time before he uses his own legs instead of a wheelchair, and his own voice instead of his mother as a spokesperson.

His capacity of vision has improved greatly and most recently the world-famous specialist for Hyperbaric Oxygen Therapy, Dr Richard Neubauer of Fort Lauderdale, Florida asked me if I was aware that Timmy is a 'living miracle?'. Isn't that wonderful?

Kira has been tested as a 'gifted child' with a very high I.Q. She has continued to grow into the most impressive, self-contained personality. The day does not have enough hours to train all her skills, and there are always new things to do — it doesn't matter if it's sports, music, painting or just talking. To raise a 'little lady' like Kira, you have to be wide-awake and functioning at 5 in the morning — added to this she is the most wonderful companion for her brother. She has a sunny personality, her sense of humour and her sensitivity brighten my day.

America has become the centre of our lives, and I have to admit that I have never felt more at home anywhere else in the world. I have made many valuable new friends.

With the help of many committed people I was able to establish *dolphin aid* in America — to support American families, and to give something back to this wonderful country. Soon we hope to have *dolphin aid* Australia up and running and the big vision of therapy centers around the world becomes clearer every day as more and more people join in.

The first German *dolphin aid* intern, Stephanie van Fallies, moved to Florida and became a full-time therapist at Dolphin Human Therapy.

Timmy's nurse Piroschka stayed in the USA and has just become the mother of a son.

Barbara, Timmy's physiotherapist, moved permanently to Florida, and has married an American attorney — Patrice is a great guy. At the time of writing she is pregnant, as well as Lerma, and nobody will believe that their babies will be born within 2 weeks of one another! Lerma too has found the love of her life in Miami.

The third Scientific Conference, initiated by *dolphin aid*, will be held at L.M.U. University of Munich in March 2003 to publish the results of the first independent scientific study about dolphin assisted therapy conducted by THE European specialist in child development, Prof. Dr Rolf Oerter — this after only 6 years of *dolphin aid* 'being in business'.

And so you see Timmy's story goes on and on, he pulls many strings in many people's lives and the answer to the question whether Timmy's accident was meant to be, to get all of this accomplished, or whether Timmy's mother tried to implant a sense into Tim's completely senseless accident, will never be answered. And at the end of the day it would not make any difference. It is good as it is, you find me as being the proud mother of two beautiful children and I am still very excited to see what tomorrow will bring.

But for sure, dear friends, I know that tomorrow will be a lot of love.

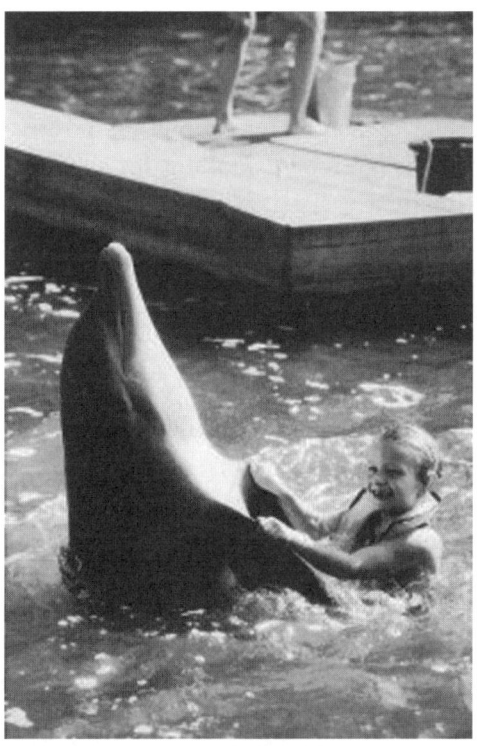

Dolphin mother and adopted child Kira

Success arises from the head AND the heart

No matter how far you go and how much you learn, there is always more to experience and more to learn. If you feel one day: 'That's it, I have got it', you can almost be sure, the next lesson is arround the corner and it will be another challenge.

When I realized that many people got positive inputs from my story and were looking for practical advice and help for their every day lives, I had to think about it for a while as it was 'all normal' for me. I grew up in a family where we experienced a lot of love, although I had to 'use my elbows' and learned not to accept NO for an answer. On the other hand, during my time owning the sponsoring agency I always had people around me who were used to being successful, be it on the side of the company sponsors, or on the side of the sportsmen, who only got sponsorships if they were successful. In trying to write down what actually helped me, I realised that by simply modelling those people during my difficult moments, I 'intuitively' did the right things which helped me to see it through.

Not all of us are so lucky to have direct contact to extremely successful people and I was asked several times during TV, Radio and Press-Interviews to share 'my secrets'. Well, there are no secrets. There are only things you do and things you don't do. And here is what I did.

Here are my personal guiding principles. They are a mix made out of values, experience and practical tips. And the best thing about them is that they are free. I received them from many other people and I am happy to share them with you.

Have a close look at them and if there is something you like, something that expresses a feeling in one sentence, a feeling you are carrying with you for a long time, feel free to use it.

That reminds me of an old Chinese fairytale, where a young man receives help from an old man and wants to return the favour of receiving help. He asks the old man what he could do for him. The old man says: 'Son, do not try to repay me. But I have one wish. Would you fulfill it?' 'Yes of course', says the young man, 'what is it'. 'Help 10 other people and ask them to do the same', said the old man.

This is what makes our world a better place and also enriches our individual lives.

My Guiding Principles:

1. You can see properly only with the heart, the essential things are invisible for the eyes.
2. Love can conquer all!
3. Only the one who continues dreaming can stand the reality.
4. Humour and courage are your strongest allies.

5. Who strives for the impossible has little competition.
6. From the stones which lie in your path, you can build bridges.
7. Those who lose courage are conquered. Winners fight on!
8. There is no situation you can change by simply accepting it.
9. Everybody has got the right to turn his own decisions upside down.

What do I exactly mean by this?

1. *You can see properly only with the heart, the essential things are invisible for the eyes*
   Use your intellect and your feeling equally. Straight in between these two, the human being has got the heart. Actions that come from the heart are always right. Follow your intuition, as its home is the heart.
   Action: Do not judge people and situations only according to what you can see with the eyes. Open yourself to feel the vibrations!

2. *Love can conquer all!*
   Love is the strongest power of all. Not only should you do things you love, but also love the things you do. Also your love will help you to create miracles. It is not only the love you feel and get from others that matters. The love you give will come back to you many times and enrich your life!

3. *Only the one who continues dreaming can stand the reality*
You can get whatever you want. You first need to dream of it, then clearly define your goals and desires to achieve it. To get to the place where you want to go, you need a destination and a map. Without these, you will get to many places, but you will never arrive at the one that makes you happy. Many people want to do 'something good', but cannot explain it in detail. If you send out the mail order 'Please deliver something nice', you can wait a long long time for the postman bringing you the parcel.

Action: Find out what you REALLY want. Imagine that your wishes 'have already become reality' — visualise your goals and desires regularly — best you do it for half an hour every day. The more you concentrate on it, the more it will manifest in your life — think of health, joy, love, and not of disease, pain and hatred.

4. *Humour and courage are your strongest allies*
Laughter is the best medicine, and joy gives rise to joy. Do not take yourself too seriously, even if you may not feel very well sometimes. It is always a matter of the perspective, and the stories of most of the children doing Dolphin Human Therapy will place your own 'problems' in the true light. Laugh about the funny things, about yourself, and about unpleasant things, too. Then you will immediately feel much better, though nothing has changed in the outside world. You ALWAYS have the choice to see either the good or the bad.

Action: Go and watch a very funny movie which you loved since you were a child. Remember situations when you had incredible fun as a child. Imagine watching these situations like 'a movie' with your mental eye. Stand in front of a mirror and give yourself a bright smile, even if you do not feel like smiling. You will always receive a smile in return — and this truth, by the way, applies on the street and everywhere else!

5. *Who strives for the impossible has little competition*
   There are no problems, unless we accept them as such. Anything is possible. Anything you can imagine can become real. As soon as you solve a challenge, the 'problem' ceases to exist for you. The more positive experiences you make, the more confident you become in mastering the situations and realising your dreams.
   Action: Continue growing all life long. Focus on your strengths and find solutions for your weaknesses. Write down your success stories, even the very little ones. This will strengthen your self-esteem and make you 'immune' to pessimists, grumblers and people who do not believe that you can achieve anything.

6. *From the stones which lie in your path, you can build bridges*
   It is up to you how you deal with the challenges (problems) you are facing, and how your story proceeds. YOU are the director of this movie, you, and nobody else, controls your life. Stones blocking

your way can stop you going further, or you can choose to use them as material to build a bridge that will enable you to pass easily above the next obstacle. Be positive and take the opportunities. Will this change the circumstances? NO. Will things resolve by themselves? NO. Will you enjoy life more and be able to have an impact on others? YES — undoubtedly.

Action: Find something good in anything that life presents to you. Start doing this immediately. Before you criticise somebody or something, first list 10 good features of this person or thing.

7. *Those who lose courage are conquered. Winners fight on!*
   Never give up, despite the difficulty.
   Action: Declare a thing that is IMPOSSIBLE TO DO to be your personal goal and work on it, until you prove that it is possible.

8. *There is no situation you can change by simply accepting it*
   Act, even if you are not sure how something works and what the consequences may be. Allow your positive thinking (desires, goals, images, values) to guide you. Many people try first to evaluate all the alternatives and their exact consequences, and therefore, they NEVER take the first step or make a decision.
   Action: Train your decision-making skills by making a small decision within 30 seconds. Almost always, you can obtain all the necessary information you need within this short period of

time, and your first feeling usually points in the right direction anyway.

9. ***Everybody has the right to turn his/her own decisions upside down***
You are allowed to change your mind any time, without racking your brains over what other people think of you. We are constantly exposed to a lot of new stimuli. If we find that earlier decisions are not right any more, we don't have to stick to them just to 'not lose face', if we have realised that they will not do any good and may even cause harm. Even if your dreams and goals remain the same all the time and you walk your way steadily towards them, you may sometimes finish up in a blind alley or on the wrong road. Then turn around and correct the course as quickly as possible.
Action: Resolve that next time you have made a decision you are not happy with, you will immediately revise it.

Exactly how does Dolphin Human Therapy work?

Over and over again people ask me why and how the 'Dolphin Therapy' functions. And shall I tell you my answer? The 'why' for me is not important, it simply doesn't matter.

The author, Antoine de Saint Exupéry said in his book *The Little Prince,* 'You can see properly only with the heart, the essential things are invisible for the eyes'. Of course I would be pleased, and deeply impressed when, at some time, science was able to produce the vitally important proof. And maybe then I would have reached the final goal of all my efforts. But until that time it is enough for me to know that the Dolphin

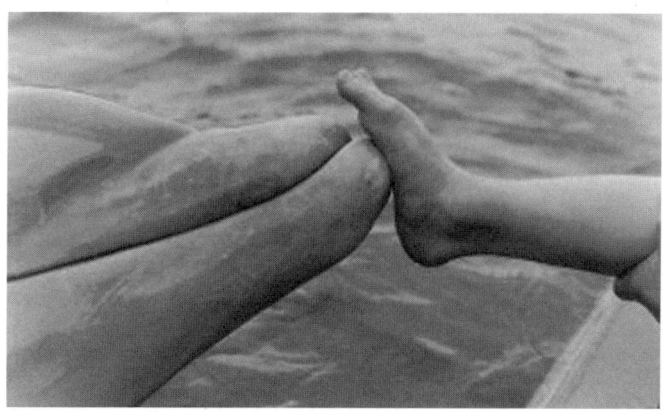

Does it matter how it works?

Therapy is much more than the question about the scientific proof of its effects. Dolphin Therapy means happiness and what more could we give a 'special needs' child than a laugh??? Lots of these special children cannot enjoy a visit to Ocean World and the Parrot or Monkey Jungle. It isn't fun for them. And for some, the wonderful Disneyland, be it in Paris or Orlando, doesn't light up their lives.

Not all 'special needs' children are happy to go to the fairground, and they can't go to the zoo. They are frightened by the loud noises and by the lights at the circus. Neither can they jump about on the playground. They cannot grip and play with model railways, or dress Barbie dolls. Dolphin Therapy is no miracle cure, and it doesn't claim to be. In the worst case a handicapped child has spent a good time with the dolphins, and is one thing — for certain — happy!!

'From the stones that lie in your path you can build bridges' a very good friend of mine said.

I hope that the reading of this book makes you part of this bridge.

***

This is my personal view and experience and I totally understand that you still want to know more about it. I have enclosed in Part 2 some specific information about Dolphin Human Therapy, more reports from other children as well as other opinions on this form of therapy. In Part 3 will you get plenty of information upon which you can start your journey. I can only encourage you to do so, you will have a great time.

II

The dolphins help many children

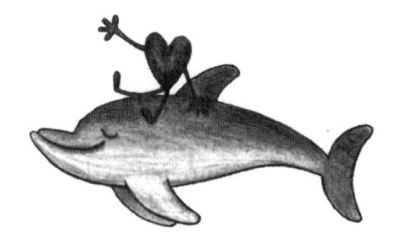

A few words from Dr David E. Nathanson

I feel honored to be able to write Kiki Kuhnert a few words and to wish this book every success. Everyone who knows me or my Dolphin Human Therapy program will also know that I only judge people by what they do and not by what they say. The best, most worthy, mission I can imagine is that to help sick or handicapped children and their families.

Kiki has helped many children and their families through the enormous efforts of *dolphin aid* and *dolphin aid America*. Her interest in these children is sincere and honest.

Her love for her son Timmy and her commitment to ensure that Timmy receives the best possible treatment are breathtaking.

Kiki is a person you really must get to know. She is that rare combination of passion and compassion which help to make this world a better place.

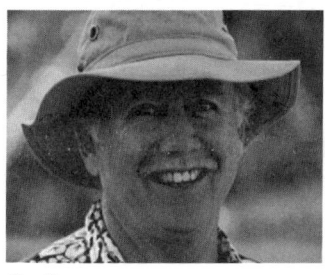

Dr David E. Nathanson
President of Dolphin
Human Therapy

Dr Dave

What is Dolphin Human Therapy?

In these days of knowledge and technology there is often no place left for miracles. In Florida and in Israel however — in the Dolphin Therapy Centers — something wonderful happens — every day.

The leading roles in these fairytales are called Alexandra, Katharina, Kristina, Tim, Lukas or Cindy. Their friends are Dingy, Spunky or Squid — Dolphins who help children.

In Dolphin Therapy Centers the children have, with the help of human therapists, games and dolphins, done things which they had never ever done before — in any previous therapy — laughed for the first time, spoken the very first word ever, or for the first time in a very long time, moved without constant spasms. The Dolphin Therapy is a program which enables children who have mental, physical and psychological difficulties to find new ways towards recovery together with their therapist and the dolphins. This extraordinary therapy method was developed by Dr David E. Nathanson, psychologist and human behaviour specialist. He is in charge of Dolphin Human Therapy and together with his wonderful team of teaching and therapeutic experts has already helped children from over fifty different countries in the world. The focus of the therapy is the coming together of the children with the dolphins. The children 'work' at appointed times on a floating dock together with their individual therapist and at least one dolphin.

The dolphin recognizes the problems which the child has and approaches in a playful and gentle manner. In this way the child loses any fears which it may have of the large animal, with whose help they rebuild contact to their surroundings and discover their self confidence. This is highly important for the children to be able to feel the impulses of the world around them, to use them and thereby to develop further. Children, whose lives were mostly lived in isolation and were ruled by apathy, show reactions. The positive influences lead to amazing steps forward in their development and have far reaching positive results. Dolphin Therapy does not claim to be a healer of any illness — but scientific studies have proved that sick and 'special needs' children, working in conjunction with dolphins, learn up to four times more quickly, and their learning process is much more intensive — and they discover their desire to explore their environment. In order to achieve the best results the Dolphin Therapy should last for at least two weeks. A further positive effect is that the families of the children receiving therapy are also drawn into the process, which also benefits the little patient's progress enormously. Also the brothers and sisters usually enjoy being in the company of the dolphins.

Dolphin Human Therapy is more than a concept. Dr David E Nathanson is the founder and the president of the Dolphin Human Therapy (DHT), Inc. A private company which provides a full time, individualized dolphin-assisted rehabilitation program for special needs children and adults.

So to begin with, it is important to not confuse the name Dolphin Human Therapy and the function of it with any other organization or group using the term dolphin therapy or dolphin-assisted therapy (there are many other expressions as well). Helping special needs children and their families should be the aim of all institutions promoting DOLPHIN THERAPY (or similar). Being the pioneers in the field of dolphin therapy, DHT can be named as the leading center and Dr Dave as the leading expert. However, there are some very serious operations and there can NOT be too many good therapy centers. Dolphin Reef in Israel and Island Dolphin Care in Florida are well known and there is a group of people working on setting up a center in Australia. It is important though to have a close look at the specific offerings of a dolphin therapy operation.

Since 1989, DHT for example has conducted over 30,000 therapy sessions representing families from 39 states and 54 countries. DHT's effectiveness is due to a simple principle — participants interact with the dolphins as a reward only after they have correctly completed their work.

Following the initial assessment and consultation with parents, the therapist develops a treatment plan to meet the needs of each child. Typically, treatment goals focus on improving speech and language, fine and gross motor skills, self-care skills, social interaction, behavior, eye contact and confidence. In addition to the team of professionals working with each child, significant parent training is an integral part of the program.

DHT has been able to help participants from all over the world. To give you some figures, over 1,400 children from the US, over 500 from the UK and even 15 children from Australia have been experiencing the Dolphin Human Therapy at DHT. Most participants have multiple diagnoses. The most common diagnoses are cerebral palsy, Down syndrome, and autism, although DHT treats all disabilities, including the severely and profoundly disabled. In addition, DHT works with children who are referred by non-profit groups and several support organizations worldwide.

The DHT program is family interactive. The staff encourages input and participation from parents, teachers, therapists, and physicians. DHT believes that family involvement, support, and follow-up is essential to the future success of special needs children and adults.

The Dolphin Human Therapy program is composed of:
- Parent orientation
- Initial parent consultation with therapists, including goals and objectives
- Review of prior therapies, records and reports
- Parent training workshops usually held three times a week.
- Daily therapy sessions including on-dock and in-water work with therapists and dolphins
- Informal meetings directly before and after every therapy session
- Professional and personalized photo album of your child's experience at DHT
- Session summaries, recommendation packets and formal written reports

Therapy is usually conducted once a day, Monday through Friday, over a period of two to four weeks. During this time, the child/adult will work with the same therapist on the goals that have been established during the initial family consultation. The therapist may consult with other staff members in planning the best treatment for the patient. Goals may include, but are not limited to, improving cognitive function, affective response, speech and language, fine and gross motor skills, self-care skills, social interaction, behavior, eye contact, and confidence.

Swimming with dolphins is a great experience and it touches almost everyone deep inside. We do not know why exactly — and maybe this will stay a secret. For healthy people it is sometimes 'just fun' and there are many places in the world one can swim with dolphins. For special needs children it is much more than swimming. Being in the water is a major relief already as the body benefits from the weightlessness and usually the children are able to move more freely. Interacting with the dolphins is a special bonus during the therapy and having experienced this once, the children gain a strong motivation to experience it again. This is the basis for very good learning progress and a lot of unexpected results. Combining the dolphin experience with a proper therapy which is based on the diagnosis seems to be the most successful way to benefit from the concept of dolphin human interaction.

A lot of scientific proof will be most likely produced in the near future and it is good that the scientists are looking for answers. There are studies being conducted currently and the results will very likely change the attitude of some representatives of the medical profession as well as of the health funds and medical insurances.

For those who have a special needs child or as adults suffering from major physical limitations, the WHY is less important than the results they experience.

As always there is the other side of the medal. Lots of activists complain about the fact that dolphins are being held in captivity for the benefit of the human beings. There are many things to say but mainly I would like to emphasise 3 facts.

First, the dolphins are used to working with their trainers and the patients. They like it very much, they are happy and that shows best in the fact that they reproduce themselves in the centres, which they usually don't do in captivity.

Second, the dolphins are held under conditions where they could escape easily by simply jumping over a 60 cm high fence and swimming away. These fences are more for the protection of the dolphins.

Third, most of the people supporting Dolphin Therapy also engage themselves for the protection of the environment and the rescue of maritime mammals. If you really want to do something for the dolphins, do not start with those few being held in special centers. One should start with those thousands of dolphins being killed every year due to greed and indifference. Find out more about them and become active.

Those children and families who have experienced a dolphin therapy are all very thankful for the existence of the dolphins and are working on giving something back.

Readers who would like to have more information about Dolphin Therapy are recommended to take a look on the Internet. Under the search-code 'Dolphin Therapy' several hundred home pages are to be found.

Comprehensive information regarding scientific work, studies on the subject are also to be found under the same search-code.[1]

Use the following links to find a great deal of comprehensive information:

http://www.dolphinaid.org
http://www.dolphinaid-oz.org
http://www.dolphinhumantherapy.com
http://www.dolphinreef.co.il
http://www.islanddolphincare.org

---

[1] Part of this text by courtesy of **Dolphin Human Therapy (DHT), Inc** - www.dolphinhumantherapy.com

How does one describe a 'dream job'?

The Therapist Marcia McMahon on her work as a Therapist:-

I work with wonderful children, and I can influence and discuss with the families the daily progress made. I experience the energetic motivation generated by the warm sea water and the dolphins. What could be more perfect?

Through a friend, who had read many articles about him, I first heard about Dr David E. Nathanson and his work. When Dr Nathanson established the Dolphin Research Center as the base for his program, I had the opportunity to get to know him and to see his work for myself. That was in May 1994. At that time the therapy offered was composed of a two-day program. The waiting list was very long.

Dr Nathanson moved to Dolphins Plus at Key Largo and I followed him. I offered my voluntary services and worked as an assistant, in the end getting the chance to become a therapist in his team.

Working with children was nothing new for me. Over fifteen years I had gathered experience from many groups of children with specific needs. But it's a very special experience to work within the framework offered by Dolphin Human Therapy. The center has an atmosphere of friendliness and peace. We work very hard, but we also work equally hard to make things happy and to build self confidence, making the learning an enjoyable experience for these kids.

It never fails to surprise people when they ask what my job is and I tell them that I work for Dolphin Human Therapy. They say 'Oh, you work with dolphins?' and I always laugh and reply 'No — I work with a whole bunch of wonderful children, the dolphins are only a part of the whole thing'. The children are the central focus of our work.

I have to admit that it's great fun to hug a dolphin, to be drawn through the water or to get a 'foot push'. But the really great challenge in this job is to get a child, filled with fears, to touch the animals or to get into the water and to be drawn alone through it for the first time by a dolphin. The laughter is worth more than a thousand words! It's just something you have to experience for yourself.

Imagine a child who has no control over his or her head, for the first time with 'head held high' following the movements of a dolphin right and then left, or one with cerebral palsy, who cannot hold on to anything, reaching out that very first time to hold the fin of a dolphin.

When someone had asked me five years ago to describe my 'dream job' I would have had no ideas. Today I am well able to answer this question.

Dolphin Human Therapy is a wonderful therapy program, carried out by a few extraordinary people and has an exceptional therapeutic base, whose guidelines have been set out by Dr Dave.

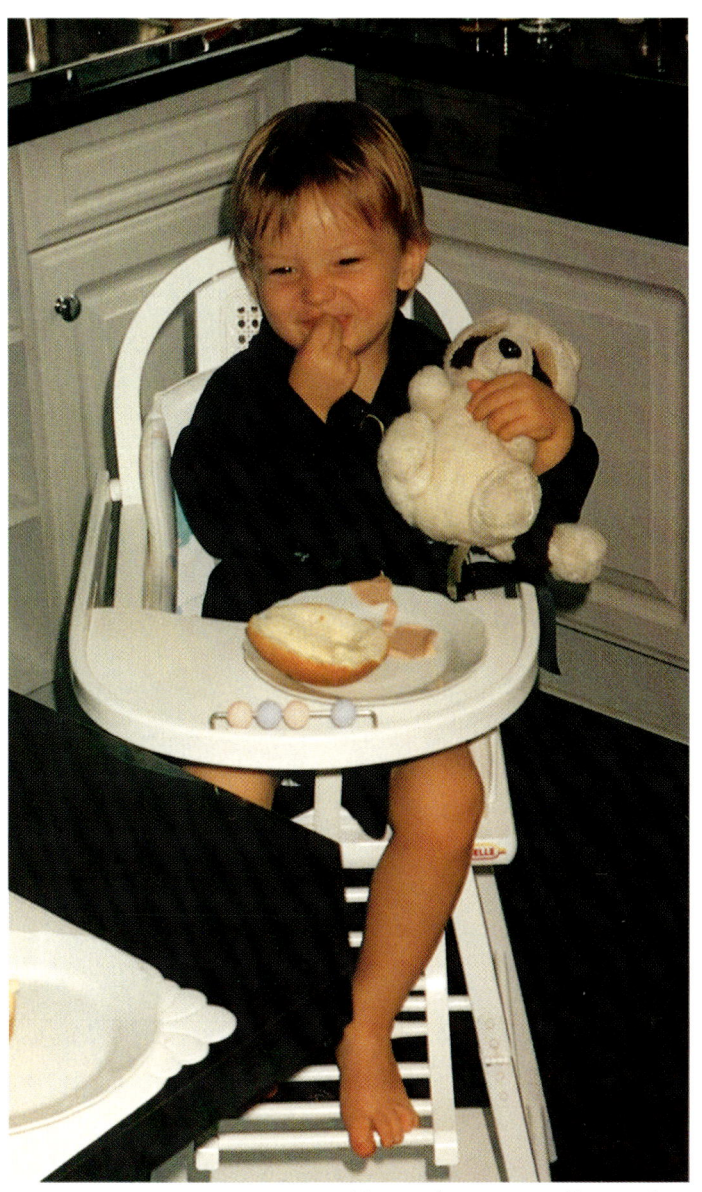

Tim on the morning of his accident

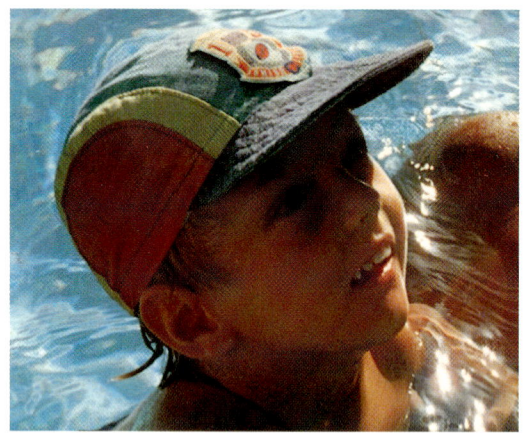

TIM'S THERAPY SUCCESSES

'Looks like I am really well'

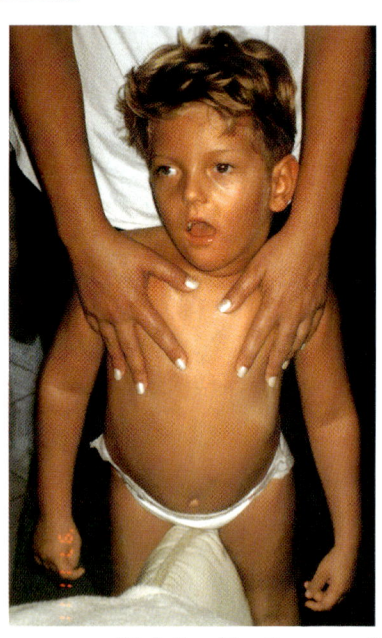

'Unbelievable - I can stand'

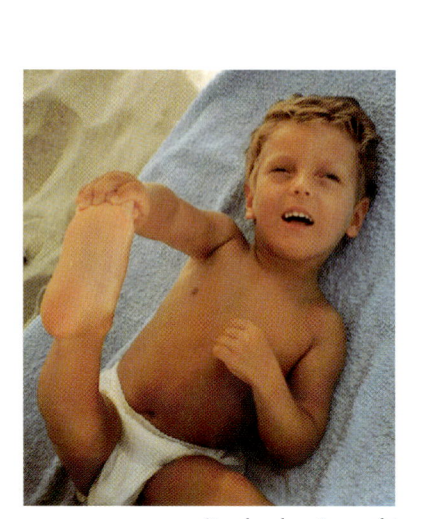

'Look what I can do'

Tim and his therapist Barbara

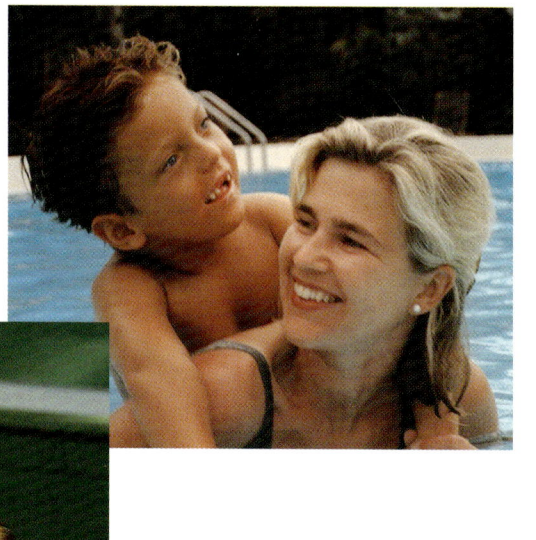

'Dolphin therapy is cool' - Tim and Michael Lauer

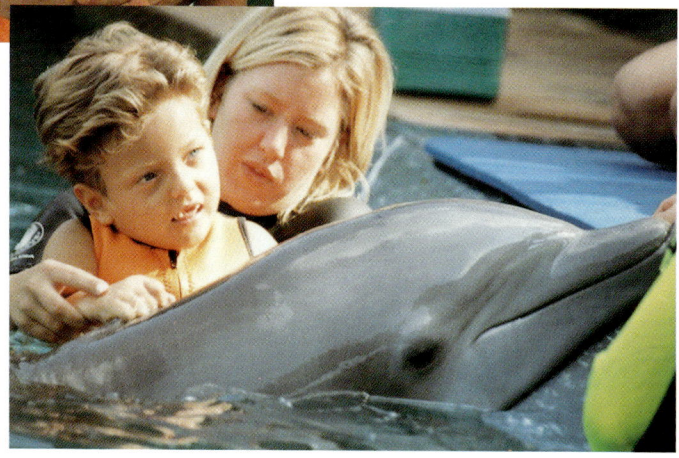

'Life is great' - Tim and therapist Heather

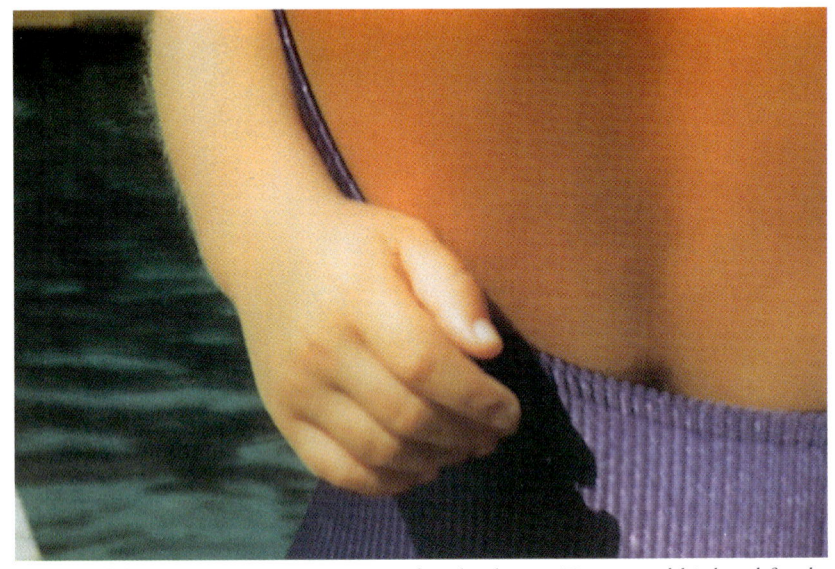

One of the most important moments: after the therapy Tim opened his hand for the first time

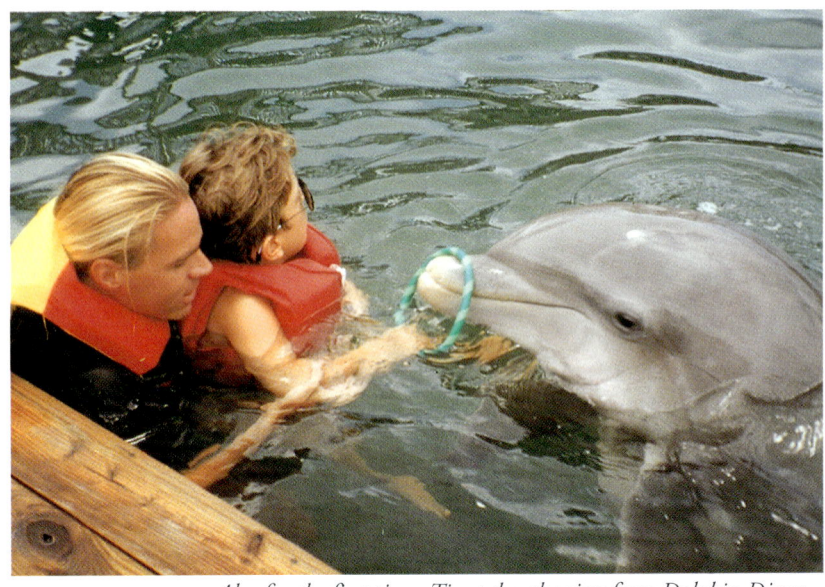

Also for the first time: Tim takes the ring from Dolphin Dingy - Dr Shannon is amazed

Dolphin therapy, a bird's-eye view

By Claudia Dichter, Journalist

At last the time has come. Here I am sitting in the aircraft heading for Miami, behind me a family from Römberg with their daughter Sina, a small child three and a half years old. She is one of six children that Stephanie von Fallois, a German Psychologist and myself, will be taking care of, as voluntary *dolphin aid* helpers during the next two weeks. Sina is suffering from 'Lupus' which is an immune syndrome. And because of this she spent the first two years of her life in hospital. At some stage she stopped accepting food. Since 1995 she has therefore, had to be tube fed, night after night she received drip feeds which contained all the necessary things in order to simply keep her alive. The hope of her parents is that with the help of Dolphin Human Therapy it may be possible to motivate Sina into eating and drinking again herself.

Dolphin Human Therapy — somehow it has a magical note in my ears. Like the majority of people I am fascinated by dolphins, these intelligent mammals, about whom so many myths and stories exist. Tales of how, in the wild, dolphins have saved people who were drowning or in danger, even protected those who were threatened by man-eating sharks. I have also heard and read much about the healing energy said to exist when handicapped children come into contact with these wonderful creatures — romantic presentations of the wonder-healer Dr Dolphin.

It's Monday morning and I am introduced to the other families. Julian is eight years old, he is there, with his family, the Bade family too, with daughter Alexandra and Kristina Lott a little girl, also accompanied by her family. I will be observing the morning session, taking care of them.

Kristina is almost four — she reminds me of St Exupéry's *The Little Prince* — she looks as if she had fallen to earth from some distant star, and didn't quite know what she was doing here. Most of the time she just holds her little hands, which are drawn into tight balls, in front of her mouth, and her eyes are very firmly shut. Together with her therapist, Heather, we go down together to the dock, for 40 minutes 'work'.

'Look into my eyes Kristina'. Heather draws the small child close to her and fixes her gaze. 'Look into my eyes.' Kristina must learn to establish eye contact. To come out of that 'sleeping beauty' state — that is the prime objective of this therapy. Since having a triple vaccination for Tetanus, Diphtheria and Polio two and a half years previously, Kristina had slowly sunk from being a normal healthy child into total apathy and, for us, a far distant state of withdrawal.

Dolphin Tori comes over to our dock and lies in the water squeaking in front of Kristina. She blinks for a second and then again closes her eyes. 'See nothing, hear nothing', that's Kristina. Over and over again Heather tries to motivate her. To look, and to reach out and touch the dolphin. These are minute steps we are talking about. The smallest impulses in the direction of movement are little successes. That, at first, I have to really first understand. Then 'hop-hop' is not the way it goes here. It's not the wonder cure — child sees dolphin, swims off for a round together and all is well. No, no, that's not the way it is.

Kristina is crying. Heather has got down into the water together with her and the dolphin to have physical contact for the first time. It's too cold for her weak and skinny body and she is shivering a little and her brow is furrowed in frustration. I feel irritation myself. Kristina is crying, the little girl that Stephanie is caring for on the dock opposite is crying too — and making noises which signal that she feels less than contentment at the sight of the dolphins.

So that's what it's like, this Dolphin Human Therapy!! ??? Where are the children speaking their first words after years of silence, those taking the first steps, or those who suddenly grasp after something out of their own initiative? Where are the mothers sobbing their eyes out for joy, unable to believe what has happened, where the fathers who are so emotional that they cannot even record it on video? I know — they are all fairy stories. But that's the way it had been written in the articles I had read.

Such figments of the imagination have to be first cast from one's mind. After my first day's observation that's quite clear to me now. The therapy is long, patient, hard work, for the children and also for the therapists.

Over and over again they have to repeat the things, motivate the children to pay attention — and to fight their stubborn wills! Handicapped 'special needs' children, especially, have a will of their own. And what a will. Real fights of strength are fought out there on those docks. Only too often I have seen the situation 'I'll cry and shout until you stop and leave me in peace'. Not here — the strong relaxed method of Heather and the other therapists is cause for sheer wonder to any observer. That of the children too.

When they have understood that working together is not such a dreadful thing, the therapist isn't 'the bad guy', and that as a reward there's this strange silvery something in the water — then the ice is broken. Sometimes it takes days, with one child maybe three, with another six or seven. But, with all who I saw, within my two weeks of observation, the breakthrough was suddenly made — at some time. And this moment always is very special. Kristina had her eyes open. She smiled at Heather and concentrated on the task of reaching for the blue ring Heather was holding up. She was breathing quickly and shivering — but this time for excitement — as she managed to grasp the ring and to hold it with both hands, she radiated absolute happiness. And proud of herself too she was! In the water also she was no longer the same child. Held firm in the arms of her therapist, the dolphin drew her through the water and she giggled just like a normal happy child. The way she looked at me when I lifted her out of the water I will never ever forget. Filled with happiness, joy, and trust. Then I almost began to cry.

Every day something new happens. The two weeks just flew past. Kristina is fully awake and attentive during her session. Sina, with no problem at all, carries out the tasks Donny asks of her. From crying and spitting like a cat from sheer rage — no longer something to be mentioned — for now she can no longer wait to get into the water.

Katherina, a seven year old little girl, suspected of being autistic, who only arrived at the weekend, suddenly starts to speak — that is one of these miracle moments, and even Alexandra who usually does her routine of crying and 'leave me in peace' habit, as stubborn as a donkey, suddenly seems to be enjoying the therapy.

A miracle? Hardly — although the key moments I witnessed during my two weeks certainly had a magic about them; all the previous hard work, effort and patience was maybe forgotten through that which just happened in the water. That's a ray of light, a little window perhaps — which gives some indication of what these children have in them, the children who so often have given up, and have been given up and dismissed by their German doctors.

A big success

Every tragedy, no matter how terrible, also has something good about it. Without Timmy's accident there would be no organization called *dolphin aid*. Without Timmy's accident hundreds of children with the most varied forms of handicap would not have had the opportunity to find a little happiness in their lives — 'a ray of sunshine' through Dolphin Human Therapy.

When in the end my son's accident still remains for me, forever, to have been completely futile, it has still left a legacy for many other children. In the past years I have been privileged to witness big and small miracles, and have cried tears of happiness as well as those of depression and sadness. Then not all children make this new start, and some didn't even have the opportunity to meet the dolphins, because God decided to call them home.

The families who took upon themselves the enormous effort and considerable burden of the trip to Florida, to make it possible for their children to meet with the dolphins, are all of one opinion about the results of the therapy. Their reactions, letters and diaries open a window into their emotional world and show how committed, strong and courageous they are in their fight, so that their children may have a life worth living.

Lukas

Take for example the seven year old Lukas. As one of the first children to take part in a *dolphin aid* journey, he brought his mother, Maria Boerner, to tears when, for the first time since his birth, he looked his mother right in the eyes and gently touched her. I remember so well Maria's state of disbelief.

Maria and her husband Michael had so longed for a child. They wished for nothing else. When Maria was pregnant with Lukas everything seemed to be perfect — luck at last. Maria enjoyed her pregnancy, up until one Wednesday, 16 October 1991, when Lukas wanted to force his way into this world. It was a very complicated birth which ended, out of the critical situation, in a caeserian section, a traumatic experience for both mother and child, as Maria told me; and she still is convinced that Lukas, with his autistic condition, is taking his revenge upon the world for this horrific experience.

When the Boerners realized that there was something wrong with their little son they were merely labeled, by the doctors at first, as being hysterical parents. And on the way, their long trail, their odyssey, was the most devastating diagnosis with which they have ever been confronted, that of a rare syndrome with a projected life expectancy of only two years.

Luckily Maria did not want to accept this diagnosis. Therefore Lukas's parents left no stone unturned when it came to trying every possible form of therapy in order to try and shake him out of the stereotyped remoteness — to try and reach him.

When Lukas was four years old his development just stagnated. The therapies no longer reached him. At about this time his mother read an article about the newly-formed organization *dolphin aid*.

In the meantime Lukas could already walk, but was most unstable on his legs, which were far too thin, and without a supportive hand he didn't want to walk at all. His mother was exhausted from all the therapy attempts, and she longed for, understandably, a significant change in the state of Lukas' health.

For Lukas still had no understanding of speech, he showed no facial gestures, he didn't speak and his physical state of health was very unstable. He could not react to any requests from his parents. Lukas sought no contact to our world and allowed no contact with his. And then he met the dolphins…

Anyone seeing this little boy today would not believe that this is the same child. Lukas is a star. He gives the wettest kisses, has the cheekiest grin, and when he meets me, looks me right in the eyes — with his, which are now full of life. The boy who, not so long ago, met us with total incomprehension is now right in the midst of us.

After the dolphins had opened the door on his world, be it just a little crack, Lukas discovered his love of my daughter Kira — for an autistic child a sensation.

Whenever Kira wanted to, he let himself be taken by the hand, danced in circles with her, and wanted to go on and on, wanted to have more and more contact, being spoken to, gentleness — and he was happy to be able to take part in things with us.

This little guy who was never able to take more than three steps alone on his spindly legs, today rocks like mad, even standing up! He laughs himself to death, in the meantime, when I tell him what a cheeky monkey he is.

Via a computer and with the assistance of sign language, he is able to communicate with his parents. He can make quite clear what he wants and Maria and Michael are very proud of this splendid chap. He still is in love with Kira. I have told him that if he wants to marry her then he will have to ask me — and that in complete sentences. I'm sure that he will manage it.

How much the dolphins changed little Lukas can only be said by his mother:

'Dolphin Human Therapy simply means everything to me — yes — for my whole family. A life worth living, joy at living and self confidence and new values. Looking back over the years 'Living with dolphin aid' has totally transformed our lives. Everything has changed.

I compare the first Dolphin Human Therapy my son took part in to a door, which opened into our world for him. The achievement of the dolphins is that our son has come closer to us. I will never ever forget how Lukas, on the last day of therapy, in the car on the way back to the hotel, kissed my hand — exactly as the dolphins do. He laughed, looked deep into my eyes — and the door was opened. How I cried.

From this point on everything went more easily. The development of my son accelerated and his understanding of us got better day by day.

Dolphin Human Therapy was, and is, for us, the key to bringing Lukas out of his world into ours. We have been able to get to know many people who have changed our lives and also changed us. Through these people I have learnt the most important thing for Lukas and myself:- that life with a 'special needs' child is beautiful, that I can be really proud of my child, and that when one confronts the world around us full of its prejudices, full of confidence, one can continue life and be happy.'

It's amazing to see how much strength and energy the parents of many sick children have. Without giving up and full of hope they continue looking for a way to help their children — irrespective how strange a therapy may seem or however difficult the chosen path may be.

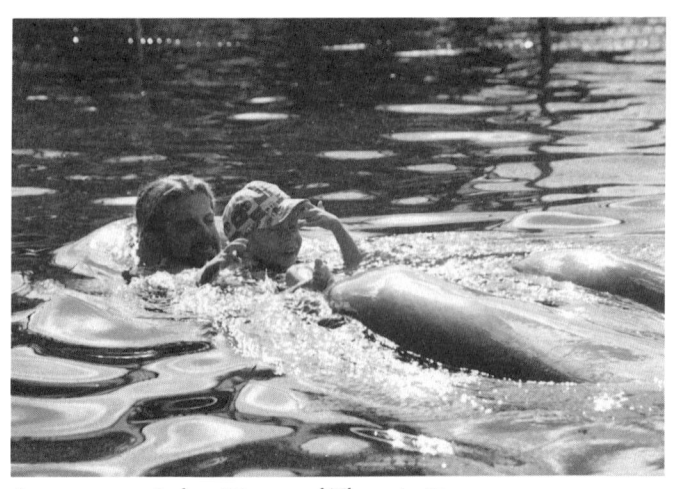

A great team - Lukas, Dingy and Therapist Donny

Katharina

The mother of nine year old Katharina, Gaby Haag-Porzel, had tried every trick in the book to help her daughter, whose condition just did not conform to any known framework, and whose symptoms in total did not make it possible for the doctors to reach a clear diagnosis. Katharina, too, is one of the stars in the '*dolphin aid* family'. Following the therapy she has developed in a more than astonishing way, as her mother proudly tells us:-

It's so difficult to put into words what the dolphin therapy means to me. Because the doctors and professors were unable to reach a clear diagnosis in the case of Katharina I had decided, at some point, to take other steps in order to try and help my child. The many therapies that were proposed in the course of the years, and did not help, didn't make treatment any easier. And so I was forced to accept, in the end, that no one could tell me exactly what was wrong with my child.

This 'other way', far from the accepted medical practice, was, at first, completely new territory for me, and I often had to fight against scorn and misunderstanding. The collective shaking of heads did not divert me from the belief that there must be a method of treatment that would really help my daughter.

I have learnt chiro-phonetics and had success with this in treating Katharina. Slowly I eased myself into a knowledge of homeopathy and found it to be a very good supporting method of treatment when employed on my daughter. And at last I came upon a fascinating method of treatment from America. The dolphin therapy.

This was a few years ago on an American cable network that I was watching by chance. I was absolutely full of enthusiasm for that which I saw. I set the idea in my head that I wanted to make that possible for my child — I will have Katharina treated there. It took many years and needed a lot of patience until, with the help of dolphin aid, *I had managed it.*

There are moments and situations that you never forget in your life. For me many of these happened during the first therapy in Florida.

The overwhelming feeling when Katharina, after the years of work and planning, for the first time, really swam with the dolphins — the day on which my daughter, for the very first time, spoke words that she had never spoken in her life before, and that she was for the first time in her life really awake and aware — the American reporter who had wanted to interview me and instead sat beside me on the steps, crying.

And of course, the magical moment, when Katharina laughed out loud the very first time — from deep inside — and really loud!

Therefore I cannot say often enough what this therapy means to Katharina and me. Courage, hope, energy and the knowledge that against all opposition I had done the right thing. I never stopped listening to my inner voice, and for that I have been richly rewarded.

Today the Dolphin Human Therapy is quite simply the best and most effective method of therapy that I can imagine for my child. It's a very expensive method, but a rewarding effort, to give Katharina the chance of a better life.

How is Katharina doing? In the meantime she speaks in complete sentences — and her speech development is coming on in leaps and bounds. It's as if she merely had a few years' delay. She now lives in our world and really enjoys it. Instructors, teachers, therapists and all our friends confirm this development. I am so proud of my little daughter and of her strong will. I am amazed at her strength, and I am proud of myself, that I managed to make this therapy possible, that I never gave up and that I always believed that we could achieve all this — and we beam this out to the world! Our life had become easier in a most particular way. I think we have taken something really important from Dolphin Human Therapy — into our hearts and into our heads. Something that no one can ever take away.

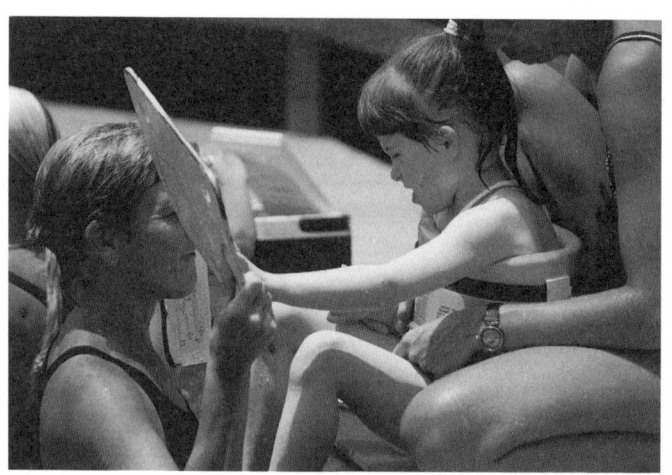

Little Katharina exercises using the 'Symbolplates'

Alexandra

Also eight year old Alexandra has taken big steps with the help of the dolphins. Her life of suffering began at the age of 13 months. Up until that time she was a normal healthy child, already able to walk, but who then deteriorated right up to the point of losing all bodily movement. After the doctors had, in the course of time, reached no firm diagnosis the parents began to search for themselves. During the search for the reason behind the condition of their daughter and the best possible help, they came upon *dolphin aid* and the Dolphin Human Therapy. This is what Claudia Bade, Alexandra's mother, has to say:-

In Alexandra's case Dolphin Therapy is the only form of therapy with which to date we have had any positive results for her development. We are still amazed at what was set free within our daughter during this short, two-week therapy. While still in Florida, at the end of the therapy we were already to confirm the first successes. Alexandra was able to sit up far better and her eye contact with others had improved, her reactions were quicker and she no longer had cold feet, she slept well and ate considerably better than at home. She enjoyed every single minute with the dolphins, she was very happy and radiated always a deep inner contentment. In the meantime we as parents have the true opinion that the pleasure and the quality of life that she experienced during the therapy are alone good reason to continue. It is absolutely a balsam for our souls to take part in this 'miracle'. Possibly the Dolphin Human Therapy is also a 'family-therapy' which is beneficial for all of us.

For me too it's a great pleasure to see how the parents of these children blossom before our eyes when they are in Florida. Anyone who has a 'special needs' child, knows the problems and distress which everyday life brings with it, how little one is able to sleep, and how much one longs for, now again, to be able to spend a few hours together with one's partner. Again and again I see how much all the parents whom I have got to know in the past years are totally absorbed in the life they are living. In Florida they suddenly notice that they have, at first with a type of bad conscience, spent a few hours relaxing on a sun bed, or perhaps have for the first time in ages been able to exchange more than just a few loving sentences with their partner. It is so important that the parents from time to time are relieved of their burden and are able to breathe in peace.

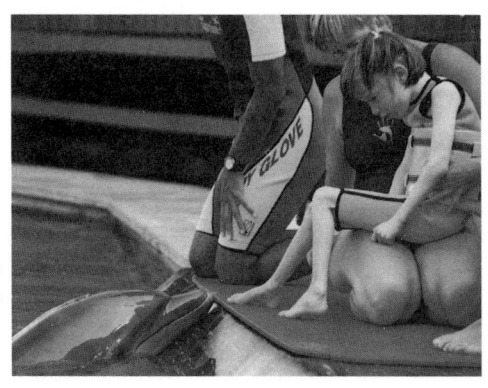

The first approach - Alexandra at the beginning of the therapy

Nadia

The parents of little Nadia, for example, had done everything imaginable to try and help their daughter. Nadia was perfectly normal and healthy at birth. But eight weeks later it became crystal clear that she was not developing normally. Compared to most of the other parents, Nadia's were not told any adventurous speculations but although no definite diagnosis could be reached, the parents felt safe in the capable hands of their doctors. Nadia's development is retarded, she is prone to cramp attacks, and her perceptive abilities are disturbed, she cannot speak and even the smallest task in daily life is difficult for her to achieve. Nadia has fully withdrawn into herself, makes no contact with her surroundings and shows a quite distinct stereotype movement pattern — all symptoms pointing to an autistic state. Bettina Haerer, Nadia's mother sums up Dolphin Human Therapy most pragmatically:-

Dr Flipper Cures Sick Children' — you can read this headline over and over again in the press. But what is this therapy really all about?

Our daughter, a child without a proper diagnosis, the doctors call it 'cerebral retardation — of unknown cause' — leaves us then always open for new things. Because she doesn't speak and is withdrawn into herself, we can only communicate with her with difficulty. My husband and I both had the same feeling when we heard of Dolphin Human Therapy — perhaps the dolphins could bring Nadia out of herself and open her up to her surroundings. Dolphins are highly intelligent animals and have a gentle way of behaving. Their presence alone has a stress-reducing effect upon humans. This we experienced for ourselves when we swam with them. The dolphins have a sonar system and are able to detect irregular frequencies. Each body has a particular frequency and resonance characteristic. In the water it is particularly easy to detect the energy field of a human. If you study the behavior of the dolphins with humans it is to be seen that they feel themselves attracted to the weak and to those who are in need of help. We saw this only too clearly with Nadia, when during the first therapy the dolphins drew her through the water with great care and thoughtfulness.

One year later during the second therapy session the dolphins asked more of Nadia. It was clear that Nadia was more confident and was able to answer this request. Even during the very first session one thing became quite clear to me. It's not just swimming with dolphins, rather a full circle. The child works on a task with the therapist. When this has been achieved satisfactorily the child is allowed into the water with the dolphins. The tasks are adjusted specifically to each child who, during the course of the whole therapy, takes steps upward. The contact with the dolphins is approached in the same manner. First the child strokes the dolphins, and then is allowed in the water where these wonderful animals gently push or pull the child through the water. The principle is quite simple:- Positive reactions are praised, brought forward and rewarded by the dolphins. A sort of behavior therapy on the 'reward' principle, the motivation for the children being the dolphins.

But not only the dolphins have this positive influence on the children. It's really the whole surrounding atmosphere, the friendly people at Dolphin Human Therapy and for a very great part the therapists themselves. They have helped Nadia with a careful, gentle, thoughtful, friendly and loving manner that came right from the heart, such that we have never, or at least seldom, experienced with German therapists. For example our therapist, Donny, came to our apartment quite outside the usual therapy times, more than once, in order to study Nadia's behavior and to discuss with us our wishes and aims. This call to duty, well above his normal therapeutic job together with his interest in the well being of our daughter, impressed us very much and he gave new advice and possibilities in dealing with our daughter. With each day of therapy Nadia became more relaxed and happier, and suddenly became aware of her own body, she began to make noises and sought contact more often with us.

Our whole family profited from our time in Florida. We became altogether much more composed and relaxed, and returned to Germany motivated and charged with positive energy. Our expectations of Dolphin Human Therapy were fulfilled. Perhaps at some point again we will have the chance to make a stop with our new friends, the dolphins, in order to recharge ourselves with 'the energy of life'.

The intensive and all-embracing counseling of the therapists, who not only take care of their little patients, but also of the whole family, forms a very important part of Dolphin Human Therapy. It is most important to be taken care of in a foreign country, where perhaps one is not able to make oneself understood easily. The long flight, the new surroundings and a foreign language — all of these things are more difficult for families with 'special needs' children. For that reason voluntary *dolphin aid* helpers as well as the therapists take great care of the parents, children and their brothers and sisters. Also the opportunity of exchanging views with other families, who have experienced a similar fate, is most helpful for the stressed parents and their children. Such exchanges, mostly in a relaxed atmosphere, can make the individual problems seem a little less huge.

All of this helps towards a successful therapy, such as can be seen from the example of Kristina.

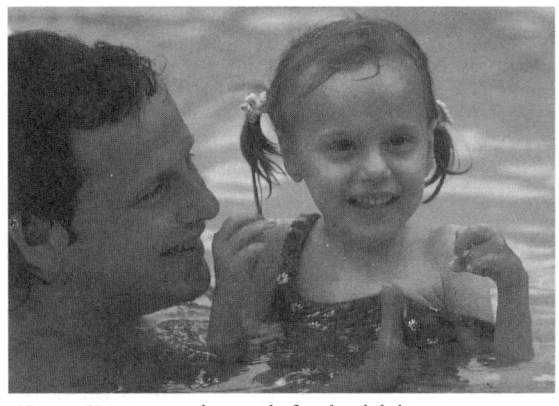

Happy Kristina - a big smile for the dolphins

Kristina

Kristina is also a '*dolphin aid* child', who was born fully healthy, and up to the age of nine and a half months quite normally developed.

Mr and Mrs Lott, Kristina's parents, pinpoint the beginning of the illness to the time of vaccination. The little girl became more and more tired and, following the third vaccination at the age of 16 months, gradually, within a period of 12 weeks became a 'special needs' child, her mother reports. She had a disturbed day and night rhythm, she slept in the daytime, but then not at all at night. She developed spastic symptoms and could no longer fix her eye-contact, and what the parents found worst of all, she no longer laughed. Also in this case the doctors could not reach any clear diagnosis. They were not able to tell the family anything further than the fact that some children, at the age of one, simply become handicapped!

Admirably the parents had the courage to have another baby, Manuel. The boy is now four years old and he is the motor and the sunshine of the whole family. Manuel has given his mother, as she says herself, back her self-confidence, because during the pregnancy with her son she had permanently asked herself what she had done wrong in the first one. Today Mrs Lott is able to look at the world again with eyes that are laughing:-

The stay in Florida was, for us all, of the utmost importance. We were able to fill up again with new energy — it was regeneration for body and soul.

The long flight to Florida went without problem from the start. I had imagined that it would be much more stressful. Each day we were welcomed by the voluntary dolphin aid *helpers and by the therapists with great warmth. The whole team is like one big family. The therapists not only take care of the children who they are in charge of, but also their brothers and sisters and of course the parents. They create a communal feeling and also one of trust. This fact was also very important and did our son Manuel good. He seeks contact with his sister far more now than in the past.*

Also the chats with the other families — on the beach, in the therapy center or during the evening meal — have also done me good, not only because of the many valuable tips and ideas, but also because I felt confirmation for myself that I had done the right thing for my daughter. Suddenly I could speak quite openly about my problems, but also about my hopes.

Kristina made great progress during the course of the therapy.

She became more concentrated, retained her eye contact with me and with others, and her hands were more often opened, she no longer had those dark circles under her eyes, she had gained weight and her whole physical state had improved. Even her hair had grown.

Leaving the dolphins, our fantastic dolphin aid *helpers and Dolphin Human Therapy fell very hard for my daughter and my whole family.*

Since our return Kristina has made further steps forward. She is growing and has gained more weight. In the meantime she can communicate better, she is happy and relaxed, and she even makes baby noises since recent times.'

At the end one particular highlight cannot be missed out, a very special, big, little miracle. Cindy's story is for me one of these wonders.

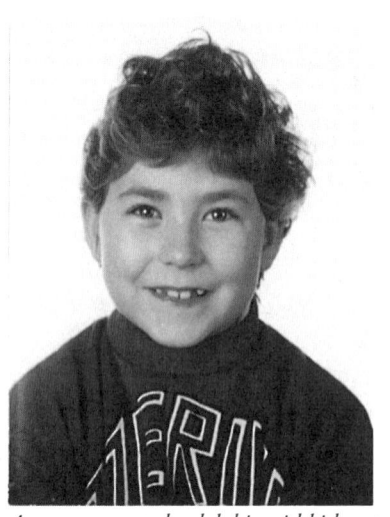

A star amongst the dolphin aid kids: Cindy has almost fully recovered from her illness

Cindy

Because of Cindy *dolphin aid* had to confront itself with a completely new mission. The call for help from her parents was received by our Wuppertal office in April 1999. Claudia Ossenschmidt called me immediately in Key Largo and told me about a little girl who was suffering from incurable cancer, and at the very most, only had a few weeks to live and had been released from a large German University hospital to die in peace. Her greatest wish was to swim with the dolphins.

Damnation I thought at first, that this should happen — it was a situation I had not thought of. What on earth were the parents going through? I began to cry. But we must, I must, *dolphin aid* must hang on in there.

Within seconds I had transformed myself into Cindy's 'undercover agent'. The average waiting time for a therapy place, even today, is about two years. It was clear that this time it had to happen quicker.

In such cases the American mentality is absolutely fantastic, a dream.

Everyone immediately recognized the situation, everyone pulled together as I ran, still sniveling, from one to the other. Half a day later I was able to report back to Germany that our 'project Cindy', with the help of Dr Dave, trainers, therapists — and of course the dolphins — could take place under the heading 'overtime'. I was so overjoyed, not three weeks later, as Cindy and her family arrived in Key Largo.

Her parents related to me the sad tale of their daughter's sickness. It must have cost unbelievable energy to endure and live with the torture that their child was going through.

In August, 1997 Cindy was examined at a University Hospital because for some time she had been suffering from a neck which was not upright — a crooked neck so to speak. This was diagnosed as being an osteosarcoma, which is an extremely evil tumor, and it was located on the 4th vertebrae of the neck. Cindy received first of all five chemotherapy treatments and in July 1998 had to face surgery on two consecutive days. During these operations she lost more blood than her poor small body had — the doctors had to twice completely replace her blood, Cindy's parents, Ludwig and Iris, told me.

The pathology laboratory examinations of the bone material showed that the tumor, on the day of the surgery, even after all the chemotherapy, had been 100% active. The stressful chemotherapies had therefore not helped at all. Even with the major surgery performed on Cindy, at three points the tumor had to remain in her neck because it would have been far too dangerous to try and remove it at these points.

At extreme high-risk. the child had to receive another four chemotherapies. And on the final examination the doctors told the family that the tumor had again begun to grow at an explosive rate, and without doubt, Cindy had therefore only a few weeks to live.

Ludwig and Iris, at the end of this treatment, had given their attention to a so-called healer. This man treated Cindy daily. He did her good. It was he who advised them strongly to try Dolphin Human Therapy — he had taken seriously the deep wish of the child to swim with the dolphins.

Cindy was certain that the dolphins would help her. She imagined that the animals, in miniature, would go through her body, swim through her blood and kill the bad cells. And therefore Barbara Schweitzer was quite surprised, the first time she was in the water with sweet little Cindy and the dolphins, to hear over and over again 'totally destroy, totally destroy'. Cindy told us herself that she meant:- 'Get out of my body you naughty bad cells'.

It was a very happy and rosy cheeked child that left Key Largo three weeks later, no comparison with the washed-out child which we knew from the beginning of the therapy. I was still heavy at heart, and dared not hope that perhaps everything would be all right. I was also so full of admiration for the family. They radiated what can only be called a total harmony. Cindy had gained weight and her hair had begun to grow. And, in her mother's words 'everything had gained', including the pleasure at life — simply everything.

In the time following I hoped to hear something from Cindy, but I was equally frightened — thinking — and what when ...? When I finally gained courage and called about four months following Cindy's departure from Florida, the parents were quite OK and Cindy was doing very well. We agreed to phone again soon with one another, and this soon turned into two more months.

During the next call Cindy's father assured me that she was doing splendidly and that her hair had grown indescribably. I wanted to ask if they had new results from a cat-scan tumorgraphy, but I didn't trust myself. But at some stage Ludwig said, almost by the way, 'The last computer tumorgraphy was really a hammer. The tumor has retarded — there's hardly anything to see, the remaining parts have encapsulated. The beast has gone into remission. What previously was tumorous material is now bone structure!.'

'Ludwig', I screamed down the phone, 'Ludwig — have you gone mad?? First of all you tell me about the hair, and half an hour later you tell me, just on the side, that the beast is in the process of disappearing?' He laughed and confirmed it all again.

Cindy is certain that the dolphins have succeeded in helping her.

The doctors at the Uni-Clinic, who dismissed her and sent her home to die, have suddenly developed a burning interest in this extraordinary little lady and recommended the parents to have extremely fine follow-up examinations done. But Ludwig and Iris have rejected this. Why should their child be exposed to all the stress again? Once a year a control check, and not more — that's all.

Next year Cindy wants to meet Dr Spunky and her colleagues once more, and *dolphin aid* will do everything it can to make this possible.

We all hope that this miracle continues, Cindy's parents are confident:-

We have asked Cindy what she especially liked about the dolphins. She said the dolphins are very loving, with beautifully smooth skin, which feels wonderful. They smell of fish and they do her good, she says. She wants to go straight back to the dolphins again, and the next time for longer. Cindy wants again to see Barbara and Brigitte, who helped her with the therapy and were so supportive.

As her mother I can only say that my child had become much more relaxed and self-confident. Since the encounter with the dolphins she has grown lots of new hair and has also gained weight. She draws a lot of dolphins and talks about them all the time. 'It was fantastic to swim with the dolphins — are Dreamer and Nicki thinking of me? — What's the time where the dolphins are? — Are they awake now?' — such questions and others come all the time.

Next year we want to do another therapy with Cindy. Hopefully we can manage it financially.

III

Addendum

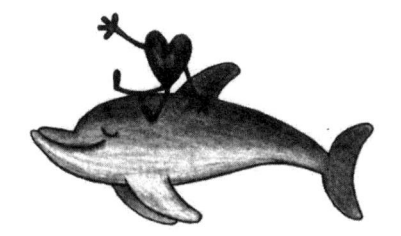

What is *dolphin aid*?

The first *dolphin aid* organisation was founded in December 1995 by Kirsten Kuhnert, who is herself the mother of a son suffering from cerebral palsy after a near drowning accident, with the intention of helping to make it possible for as many 'special needs' children and their families as possible to realize a hope-filled Dolphin Human Therapy.

Following this basic idea, the *dolphin aid* team tries with very much application and hard work, and a never diminishing enthusiasm, to achieve the aims of the charity. All members follow various professions daily and give their free time, holidays and also their private freedom happily in the never ending fight and in the service of children.

In the course of over seven years *dolphin aid* has been able to achieve much.

Today the charity helps:
- with the production, publication and dispatch of information material
- with the counseling of parents seeking help
- in arranging consultations and talks between the therapists and the parents and children
- in helping to obtain therapy places
- in helping to obtain reduced rates for hire cars and accommodation

- offering care and assistance in other countries and overseas
- offering assistance with legal and tax matters.

Until we have reached all our aims there is a long path to be taken. For it is a path we must take together with the children, and we shall take it together with parents, helpers, sponsors and donors happily.

In the allocation of the, alas, few therapy places *dolphin aid* can only be of help, because *dolphin aid* is itself not the operator.

We are sure, that in the not too distant future, it will be possible for us to realize the full spectrum of counseling, the medical and the therapeutic preparations, together with the follow-ups, the psychological attendance (also during the journeys), the research necessary to obtain the acceptance by the medical insurance companies, right through to increased therapy possibilities.

All active members of *dolphin aid* are, without exception, voluntary, do their work on an honorary basis and all work together towards the aims we have set ourselves.

We have been able to help many and we hope also in the future, to help efficiently, with those seeking help in mind, wherever possible quickly, and without bureaucracy.

Our visions can become reality every day through the hard work of innovative people. There is still a lot of work ahead of us!

To date the following organisations relating directly to the *dolphin aid* concept exist:

dolphin aid e.V. — Germany
Founded in 1995 by Kirsten Kuhnert — a charity with the aim of supporting and helping German families to achieve Dolphin Therapy for their 'special needs' children.
http://www.dolphin-aid.net

dolphin aid America inc. — United States of America
Founded in 1999 by Kirsten Kuhnert — a charitable and non-profit making organization, with the aim of supporting and helping American families to achieve Dolphin Therapy for their 'special needs' children.
http://www.dolphinaid.org

dolphin aid Australia — Australia
Founded in 2002 by Sylvia and Christian Uhrig and at the time of printing in the process of achieving the status of a charitable and non-profit making organization, with the aim of supporting and helping Australian families to achieve Dolphin Therapy for their 'special needs' children.
http://www.dolphinaid-oz.org

dolphin aid is thankful for every kind of support and totally relies on donations. Please become a supporting member in the country you prefer and donate to the organisation of your choice. Thank you!

The aims of the Charity

- to find sponsors
- to call for donations
- to support and help families with 'special needs' children to achieve therapy
- to help to make it possible
- to assist with all travel preparations necessary
- to undertake required bookings
- to accompany, to help and support with the journey (Escort)
- to offer help, support and assistance at therapy centers and facilities
- to help with the whole concept of the undertaking, paperwork, forms and other matters
- to strive to achieve the recognition of this therapy form (Dolphin Therapy) by the health authorities, health funds, medical funds
- to create and found non-profit therapy and research centers
- to give financial support wherever necessary

The therapy centres

Dolphin Human Therapy, Key Largo, Florida
http://www.dolphinhumantherapy.com

Dolphin Human Therapy is under the direction of the psychologist and human behavioral expert Dr David E. Nathanson, who for more than twenty years has been working with sick and 'special needs' children.

Dr Nathanson is really the founding member of Dolphin Therapy World, which helps extremely sick children not able to be helped by classical methods, and sometimes rejected by other centers, to a start in a better life. Infants, children and youngsters are given here, even in the light of the worst difficulties, a new quality of life. There is no minimal requirement.

Dolphin Reef, Eilat, Israel
http://www.dolphinreef.co.il

Dolphin Therapy under the direction of Maya Zilber.

Dolphin Reef in Eilat has existed now for more than 9 years. The dolphins live in the open sea and work in the day time in a large netted-off area.

The program is carried out by trained specialists including psychological support. As a result of the accumulated experience a preference is given to children with Down Syndrome, autistic children and mentally handicapped children. The minimum requirement is that the child is seven.

Island Dolphin Care, Key Largo, Florida
http://www.islanddolphincare.org
Dolphin Assisted Recreational Program under the direction of Deena Hoagland. Following successful work in the 'classroom' and on the 'platform' on the dolphin basin the children are rewarded with a swim with the dolphins. Deena Hoagland names herself to be specialized in the field of autistic children, those with behavior problems, those who have been abused and maltreated. The minimal requirement here is that the child is three years old, can control the head and is free of any seizures. The meeting with dolphins is also possible for the general public, at the individual centers. It is possible to swim with the dolphins at some centres.

Glossary

Dolphin Human Therapy
A therapy program founded by Dr David E. Nathanson (Miami), the man who conceived Dolphin Human Therapy.

Dolphins Plus
A dolphin resort belonging to the family Borguss and located in Key Largo, Florida. The home of Dingy and Fonzie — one of the most successful Dolphin Therapy Centers in respect of breeding.

Dolphins Cove
A dolphin station on the US Highway 1 — also belongs to the Borguss family. Is principally used to give a wide section of the public the opportunity to swim with dolphins. This is the new home of Dolphin Human Therapy.

Dolphin Research Center
This was the starting point for Dolphin Human Therapy. It was here that Dr Nathanson began with the first constant Dolphin Therapy. Today this is a research center, open to the public. It is also the 'old peoples home' for dolphins. Various therapy programs are in planning. The center is located at Grassey Key.

Some helpful addresses for the parents of sick and 'special needs' children

Center for Child Development
Dr. med. Inge Flehmig
Rümker Strasse 15-17
D-22307 Hamburg (Fed. Rep. of Germany)

Meike Weitemeier
Barmbeker Str. 9a
D-22303 Hamburg (Fed. Rep. of Germany)
Physiotherapist especially concentrating in the field of handicapped/'special needs' children.

St Briavels Center for Child Development
Dixton Road
Monmouth
Gwent NP5 3PR
Wales
Great Britain
An institute for child development, the therapy is geared to the Doman and Delcato methods. Founded more than 20 years ago by parents of affected children.

Dr Ramon A. Guevara
240 Crandon Boulevard
Suite 106
Key Biscayne, Florida 33149, USA

Dr Cheryl L. Butz
Marschallstrasse 11
D-80802 Munich (Fed. Rep. of Germany)
A specialist doctor for children's medicine — treatment when necessary under anaesthetic, own Dept of Anaesthetics

Prof. Brucker
University of Miami
School of Medicines
Dept of Orthopedics and Rehabilitation
Jackson Memorial Hospital
P.O. Box 01690
Miami, Florida 33101, USA
Biofeedback laboratory, functional electronic stimulation program

Dr William H. Stager
North Flageler Drive
Suite 101B
West Palm Beach, Florida 33407, USA
Osteopathic, cranio-sacral therapies and acupuncture

Richard A. Neubauer, M.D.
4001 Ocean Drive Suite 105
Lauderdale by the Sea, Florida 33308
Center for Hyperbaric Oxygen Therapy.
Dr Neubauer is a world famous expert in this field

All the above mentioned doctors, therapists and institutions have been personally tested by Timmy and found to be simply wonderful.

My thanks

Every Day a Little Miracle is the title of this book. That it has been written at all is a little miracle. In all the long nights in which Timmy directed my pen, and with every single word which has been written, this wonder has become clear to me.

My son is alive and he has set something fantastic in motion. At some time the scientific proof of success of Dolphin Therapy will be laid in writing, open for all to see. Until then a lot of water will pass under the bridge. Thanks to Timmy, who guided and inspired us to found *dolphin aid*, children will return from their visits to Spunky, Duke, Jeannie, Alfons and the other swimming therapists — every year, every month, every week and every day. And they will be able to say: Life is beautiful.

They will win for themselves trust in their own abilities, they will have strengthened the trust which they have in their parents. Whole families will be able to set off along new paths, thanks to the therapy developed by Dr David Nathanson.

I am thankful to my son that he has enriched my whole life through the task he set me, and I am also aware of how many people to whom I owe my thanks.

They had no idea that on 18 June 1994, a little two year old boy would inspire them all to think anew, and very deeply. But they have all understood. Tim's bequest is that it has brought them closer to, and given them a closer understanding of, 'special needs' children and opened their eyes and hearts to their needs.

My thanks go to:

Elke Coburger, Volker Nielsen, Inge Nielsen, Edith Evers, Helene Hüllen, Martin Schata, Albert Hornfeck, Heribert Kuhnert, Irmtraud Kuhnert, Kay Evers, Helga Evers, Hilde Elias, Martin Terhardt, Jo Struchtrupp, Els Struchtrupp, Bernhard Ibach, Michael Mandl, Bernd Appolt, Hartmuth Morgenroth, Tatjana Schläth, Rainer Pietschmann, Peter Welbers, Cathy Monceaux, Elisabeth Menzen, Adolfo, Sabine Maaßen, Alexandra Fritz, Jörg Immendorf, Hanjo Hillmann, Sabine Schwarzer, Regina Goldlücke, Hans-Joachim Stuck, Max Schneider, Michael Kneissler, Celia Tremper, Claudia Dichter, Alexander Schneider, Vera Schneider, Stefan Müller, Johannes Riemann, Walter Blum, Andrea Müller, Oliver Schielein, Ulli Richter, Phillip Schneider, Michael Eschmann, Karin Weißflog, Katharina Schneider, Reinhard Maßberg, Gabi Richter, Jaqueline Schierl, Ottmar Alt, Christian Broden, Thomas Schierl, Günther Frauenkron, Kalle Hansen, Anja Krugmann, Sylvia Waden, Jürgen Barth, Birgit Lechtermann, Petra Morawietz, Jürgen Pippig, Willy Knupp, Dieter Hahn, Dietrich Ernst, Katja Ernst, Eckard Bittner, Jan Strohmenger, Gabriele von Rosseck, Bernd Sommer, Heinz Westen, Peter Frankhauser, Petra Simon, Peter

Haslebacher, Marco Dadomo, Petra Hunold, Nicola Hipp, Lionel von dem Knesebeck, Bettina Heyne, Stephanie Ehrenschwendner, Karin Frankhauser, pro art, Antonio Pelle, BMZ, Rolf Milser, Peter Thorsten Schulz, Klaus Heer, Claudia Ossenschmidt, Janina Sorkale, Felicitas Großhans, Arnold Müller, Stefanie von Fallois, Matthias Heimer, Thorsten von der Heyde, Romeo Horvart, Brigitte Nielsen, Justin Bell, Tom Baur, Fred Woodbridge, Barbara Schweitzer, Nickel Gösecke, Franz Carpraro, Veronica Cervera, Ramon Guevara, Bill Stager, Lloyd Borguss, Annemarie Borguss, Rudolf Jäckle, Heidrun Tackenberg, Manuela Tarnowskij, Meredith Mesa, Gerti Kleikamp, Stefan Schneider, Meike Weitemeier, Patrick Lindner, Markus Tedeskino, Margarete Schreinemakers, Krista Keßler-Brück, Alicia König, Petra Schuppe, Sam Shore, Michael de Shay, Kerstin Fricke, Nomi Baumgartl, Ulla Jacobs, Kuno Nensel, Boris Brand, Dirk Müller-Liebenau, Andrea Bohling, Mary Lycan, Alexandra Phillips, Peter Rust, David Nathanson, Diane Sandeline, Gitti Rust, Donny de Castro, Klaus Ostendorf, Frank Ostendorf, Marcia McMahon, Christina Collins, Lynn Cermak, Heather Friend-Nixon, Lou Ellen Klints, Arthur Cooper, Bill Shannon, Deena Hoagland, Kathy Romano, Ursula Felger, Ulrich Niese, Horst Esdar, Ulli Upietz, Monika Wasel, Christa Green, Marc Cabrera, Roswitha Rauh, Gereth Vye, Rolf Seelmann-Eggebrecht, Leontine Graefin von Schmettow, Joachim Winkelhock, Thomas Winkelhock, Frank Schmickler, Joan Mehew, Brigitte Rey, Erich Borguss, Laurie Borguss, Thorsten Schlorf, Niki Davis, Rick Borguss, Volker Riech, Tanja Guess,

Ulf Schoenefeld, Gabriel Garcia Hartmann, Reinhard Freese, Alexandra Stritt, Robert Niemann, Sarah Hutchings, Marc Pasteur, Ingrid Post, Uwe Post, Bjoern, Ina, Pia, Mats, Silke Feussner, André Rademacher, Markus Oestreich, Kris Nissen, Leslie von Wangenheim, Axel Windgassen, Hans-Werner Rosenfeld, Lerma Windgassen, Ronald Schloesser, Detlev von Wangenheim, Dagmar Rosenstein, Piroschka Kaiser, Jaqueline Nicholl Mc-Neil, S.K.H. Prinz Leopold von Bayern, I.K.H. Prinzessin Ursula von Bayern, Beate Matuschewski, Claudia Oberwinter, Tanja von der Brueggen, Tanja Pfaffenbach, Edmund Krix, Katharina Engelmann, Madu Mehta, die LTU-Belegschaft zu Luft und zu Boden, Laura Yanes, Nicole Fehr, Rita Neubauer, Wilhelm Horkel, Heiner Biedermann and Crew, Horst Salzmann, Schwester Susanne, Ilka Mantzel, Bernhard Brucker, Joachim Tomesch, die Belegschaft der Grossbaeckerei Wendeln, Stefan Klein, Ein Herz fuer Kinder, Anke Invaldson, Hildegard Ledle, Susanne Vetter, Ingeborg Lamberti, Isolde Holderied, Ralf Kelleners, Hans Bernd Kamps, Peter Sydow, Diane Demskey, Rosita Michael, Kiki Lombardi, Yvonne, Weiner, Peter Freymuth, Joanne Rose, Mayra Lecusay, Petra Sawusch, S. Makrigiani, Ulrike Ruessmann, Trudi Huppertz, Iris Gericke, Anke Ingvaldson, Hans-Gerd Lenard, Michael Schnuermann, Barbara Rosier, Daniela Hedermann, Silke Reisewitz, Sarah Harneid, Heike Heckmann, Sabine Liske-Stecher, Jochen Berninghaus, Iris Diop, Tibor Gabli, Arno Nell, Joerg Massenheim, Karl-Heinz Mutz, K I der Remscheider Kinderklinik, Dirk Morgenstern, Mirja Lullic, Britta Lassmann, Catrin Nagel, Kathrin Bienefeld, Daniela Dustmann, Heide

Rademacher, Eberhard Maier, Christiane Pfeifer, Antje Witthopf, Birgit Brandes, Birgit Puechner, Meike Wrede, Ingela Rust, Evamaria Bienel, Heike Gede, Alexa Mersch, Catja Mersch, Henning Lohse-Busch, Knut Krecker, Kirsten Kramer, Fury in the Slaughterhouse, band ohne namen, Reamonn, Liquido, Naima, The King, Alternative Allstars, Chumbawamba, Brings, Glow, Somersault, Natural Born Hippies, Martin Schenkel, Score!, Gotthard, Andrés Ballinas, Peter Maffay, Katy Karrenbauer, 2raumwohnung, Wonderwall, Worlds Apart, Badesalz, Münchner Freiheit, Purple Schulz, Wolf Maahn, Christian Wunderlich, Bläck Fööss, Samer Nassif, Elias, Dankner, Beam & Yanou feat Domenik, Thomas Anders, Irena und die Regenbogenkids, Rosemary Keating, Dee Light, Yvonne Nelson, Silvia Uhrig, Michael Kent, Terry Hill, David Green, Lizz Boardman, Jürgen Obermann, Iwana & David Troughton, Sebastian Rothe, Sheldon and Maria Lowe, Linda and Robert Bailey, Susanna and Roger Khouri, Tiz Stockton, Marc, Scott, Marc Funnen, Monika Boehm, Ralf Moeller, Barbara Becker, Andrea Sabat, Claudine Wilde, Uwe Muth, Jochen Malmsheimer, Renate Castan, Jim and Betty McManus, Jürgen Eisermann,Volker and Erin Anding, Paula and Jack Levine, Anna and Guillermo Freixas, Lotta Haubold, Britta Hecker, Christina and George Lindemann, Hanta and Staertzel, Dave Maraj, Alexander Reus, Johanna Seuss, Stefan Seuss.

Thanks also to all of those whose names I may have forgotten to record here.

❖❖❖

Nomi Baumgartl

Born 1950 in Southern Germany, Nomi studied visual communication and design. She is a freelance photographer who lives and works in Munich, Germany and Maui, Hawaii.

Areas of work:
- International photographic journalism, numerous publications in magazines, books, photographic volumes
- Advertising and image advertising
- Various book projects and documentary films about contemporary artists and personalities.

For the charity organisation 'dolphin aid e.V.' and 'dolphin aid America' she has created an exceptional art work concept including a high class image campaign, exhibitions, art work calendars and media presence. International stars such as Tatjana Patitz swam with dolphins to support dolphin aid to enable dolphin therapies for 'special needs' children.
http://www.I-WONDER-NOMI.com

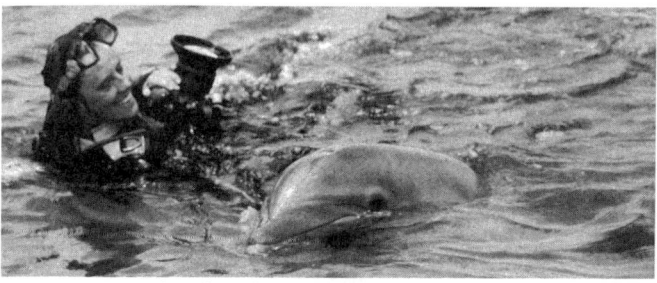

Nomi Baumgartl and Cayla« – dolphin aid project – Grand Bahama Island 2001. Photo courtesy Constanze Wild.